Dancing With Death
Thru Senility Into
Eternality

Dancing With Death Thru Senility Into Eternality

Toni Delgado

Writers Club Press

San Jose New York Lincoln Shanghai

Dancing With Death Thru Senility Into Eternality

Writers Club Press
an imprint of iUniverse, Inc.

For information address:
iUniverse, Inc.
5220 S. 16th St., Suite 200
Lincoln, NE 68512
www.iuniverse.com

ISBN: 0-595-24442-4

Printed in the United States of America

"Can you take it away? Can you kiss it away?
Maybe I am the mirror that reflects all.

When there is doubt, there is hope.
When there is fear, there is love.
When there is hate, there is peace.
When there is suffering, there is the dance.
The dance, a dance, a dance of love.
I dance to dance. I dance the Dance."

Robert Mirabal
Taos Pueblo
Music from a Painted Cave

I lovingly and gratefully dedicate this book to
my saint of a husband
Dr. Kelley Elkins,
and
To all those precious folks consciously going thru senility
and to all their caretakers

*"AN ORGANISM THAT CAN FULLY HEAL ITSELF IS
TECHNICALLY IMMORTAL"*
—Dr. M.T. Morter Jr., <u>The Healing Field</u>

Contents

ACKNOWLEDGEMENTS

I am eternally grateful for my connection to Babaji of Hairakhan, for his guidance, patience and enduring love. I am truly grateful for the many connections I have to Mother-Father God of Whom there are many aspects in the One.

I am grateful to have created a relationship with my tough as nails and gentle as giggles, life partner, Kelley Guy Elkins. Thanks Kel for being the best husband, companion, cook, baker, hair washer and comber, chauffeur, caretaker, process facilitator, cheerleader and doctor. Above all else, thanks for not giving up.

Thank you Leonard Orr for all the incredible effort you have put into the Rebirthing Movement continuously for the last 30 years, for staying in enthusiasm in your process, for loving yourself, God, Isabelle and humanity as much as you do. Thank you for teaching me about surviving senility and Physical Immortality. Thank you Isabelle, my loving sister, for supporting Leonard and the Rebirthing Movement in the high way that you do.

Thank you Jim Dvorak and Mary Bryne for the magnificent job that you did in showing me my reflections, for your impeccability as nagual teachers and warriors, and for the work you do to support those students fortunate enough to be in your presence.

Thank you Kali Mai Thompson for your patience and willingness to teach me when I was so asleep. You are indeed a great Kali.

Thank you to Dr. Richard Schulze for the masterful formulas you have put together to teach people that it is easy to caretake their bodies and regenerate virtually all dis-eases known to man.

Thank you Dr. Ron Mitchell for your continuous generosity and support in working with Kelley and me over these last few years. Your loving intervention with the Thompson chiropractic technique was and continues to be an incredible boon to our welfare.

Thank you Lucy Aristizabal, Uma Fay and Mark Patterson for your loving support over the past few years, for your willingness to process your stuff and persistence in growing into your seeds of Greatness.

PREFACE

We have wandered so far from our Beginnings that few of us have memory of who we are or why we are here. We have become so disconnected from our Source, ourselves, each other and this very precious planet that houses and sustains us. We have, in essence lost touch with our very nature.

We are (and have been for a while) in a process of redefinition...we are redefining who we are and recalling ourselves back to our Natural Created State of Divinity. When we remember enough of ourselves, we will no longer be plagued by our limitations of the earthplane. There will no longer be misery, suffering, pain, poverty, dis-ease, aging, death. We will have Heaven on Earth.

Until we arrive at that place of enoughness; until we have championed the conditioning of the programs we volunteered to heal; until we have received enough Cosmic dispensations from the Company of Heaven to speed our evolutionary and Ascensionary process; until Lightworkers have done enough selfless service to raise this sweet Earth out of the quagmire of human miscreations, we have work to do.

Mahavatar Babaji of Hairakhan said, "As long as you are in body, you have work to do". He also said that the highest form of yoga in this age—the transition between the Kali Yuga (the age of darkness) and the Sat Yuga (the age of enlightenment) is Karma Yoga. Karma Yoga is taking action-doing work, which Babaji says is also the highest form of worship.

I can think of no finer selfless service, no finer Karma Yoga than doing the work to return to the natural state that God-Goddess intended for us. That natural state is the state of Life Everlasting...Life Eternal...Physical Immortality. It is an awesome journey, reclaiming this gift and..."getting there" is packed with challenge. It is a journey worth doing. We must do it—at the very least, some of us must do it, so that it can become commonplace once again...so that others can remember.

In Satprem's <u>On The Way To Supermanhood</u> , he very beautifully writes the following: "If our natural does not become truer, no amount of supernatural will remedy it; if our inner dwelling is ugly, no miraculous crystal will ever brighten our day, no fruit will quench our thirst. Unless Paradise is established on Earth, it will never be anywhere. For we take ourselves everywhere we go, even into death, and so long as this stupid second is not filled with Heaven, no eternity will be lit with any star. The transmutation must take place in the body and in every day life; otherwise no gold will ever glitter, here or anywhere else, for ages of ages.

What matters is not to see in pink or green or gold, but to see the truth of the world which is so much more marvelous than any paradise, artificial or not, because this Earth, this very small Earth among millions of planets is the experimental site where the supreme Truth of all the worlds has chosen to incarnate in what seems to be its very contradiction and by virtue of this very contradiction, to become all light in darkness, all breadth in narrowness, immortality in death and living plenitude in each atom at each instant". (pp.74-75)

What follows are the pages of recounting my journey to Truth—to My Natural Truth through the passageways of senility and death.

INTRODUCTION

Death is number 4 on the list of fears that Americans hold. Number 1 is fear of being terrorized by terrorists (from the Commission of Terrorism 2001). Number 2 is fear of public speaking and number 3 is dread of holocaust. Most of us keep death or rather the thought of death at bay in our day to day lives, allowing it only with the periodic passing of a loved one. We don't let it consciously touch us, even though it is presented on the news daily...unless it involves a public figure we allowed ourselves to get close to like Princess Di or unless it strikes thousands of our own numbers as in the World Trade Center.

We have been acculturated in western society to accept death as the completion of a cycle; as a foregone conclusion to life and living. Religions have contributed to this belief system...so much so that the clergy have enrolled people into believing that the only way a person can achieve Heaven is to rot their bodies and drop them off.

I believe that we cannot be fully alive if we have no consciousness or understanding of what both life and death offer us. Until we immerse ourselves in the philosophies, psychologies and even perhaps the physiologies of both the life urge and the death urge, we cannot know of what we seek; we cannot make intelligent and conscious choices for ourselves for the present or for the future.

An "urge" is an impulse toward a goal. Thus a "life urge" would be an impulse toward aliveness, living and life, while "death urge" would be an impulse toward dying and death. Both the life urge and death urge are forces or energies that pulse within us. We have had a lot of experiences with both and our body-mind remembers. This is true whether you believe in reincarnation or not. Your DNA did not come to you clean of the memories from all your relations. Whether we are aware of it or not, everything from them and your past is stored within you.

The quality and quantity of what is stored about life urge and death urge absolutely affect our daily lives moment to moment. It only makes sense that the more thoughts, emotions, feelings and experiences we have on file that speak to joy, satisfaction and ease (associated with life urge), the more supported, lively and healthy will be our body-mind and our perspective on life. This then reinforces and reflects in wellbeing.

The more struggle, suffering, belief and participation with hardship, victim consciousness and punishment (associated with death urge), the more difficulty and misery we perceive that life is. With this as programming-with this as habit, we are reinforced with degeneration, illness and eventually death.

The curious thing though, is that most of us are not awake enough to recognize our patterns and our conditioning. I did wake up , however. Maybe it was my destiny that I remember or maybe it is just that I was willing to do the work to remember. Satprem says "Actually we do not seek, we are sought. We do not call, we are called. We grope about only as long as we want to do everything ourselves. There is nothing to do. There is everything to undo". (Supermanhood, p. 84) So maybe I was called to do this.

Senility is thought of as a very serious passage into death. In our contemporary worldview—in ordinary reality, senility is the precursor to death. It is what happens to folks who become aged, decrepid and useless to society and themselves. There is no survival here, because there is no consciousness about surviving it.

Senility from the perspective of an individual who has prepared for it consciously, however, is a very different experience. Senility, for this latter individual, is an altered state of consciousness, which when accepted as a phenomenal opportunity, becomes a school of learning that leads to Physical Immortality and Life Everlasting.

1) THE UNNATURALNESS OF OUR LIVES

Humanity has not existed in its natural state for a long time—for millenia. It does not remember what its natural state is because of the disconnect from Source. This state of affairs has disconnected us from everything and everyone—the Earth, our bodies and each other. It has created within us an impersonalness with regard to all our relationships. The separation is not real and yet it seems real, because we do not remember what was/is real for us. We remember nothing of our true beginnings. As a result of this "amnesia", man's idea of "natural" is stuckness in abnormalcy.

Consider, for example, the deplorable ways man has treated Mother Earth. He has polluted the airways, the waterways, and the soil. He has overused chemistry, toxifying and depleting the nutritive value of most food sources. He has created genetically modified foods (and it will be a few more years before we learn what the consequences of this will be).

He has gone against nature to create ways to produce and harness energy to accomodate his lifestyle; nuclear power plants create dangerous toxic waste that cannot properly be disposed of. He has laid waste to mountain tops, greedily scooping out coal, displacing whole communities and contaminating waterways. He is also draining the Earth of the blood within her veins—he is shameless in his consumption of Mother's vital oil.

People have refused to unite in agreement with regard to global warming; that man has in any way induced this disastrous state when many researchers have given credibility to the fact that consumption of oil, gas and coal are creating a greenhouse effect. The people who care enough to have done the research, say "if this is not addressed dramatically in the next 100 years, the Earth's temperature could raise as much as 5 degrees Celsius which would have huge ramifications for peoples around the world". (Dr. Watson, ex-Director of IPCC. Dr. Watson is the ex-director only because he is pro Earth). Man has gone against his nature here and seems to have no clue of his partnership nor his dependence on the Earth nor the consequences of his recklessness.

Consider that man is as abusive with himself as he is with the Earth. Consider the average eating and drinking habits (junk food and fast food chains plague the world). Consider that most Americans reach for a soda or diet soda rather than water (dialysis is happening younger and younger all the time). Consider that 50% of Americans are now overweight and heading to obesity. Consider that physical education is no longer part of the curriculum in many schools.

Consider that America spends over $500 million dollars yearly in laxatives to ease their constipation. (The effects of long term constipation are causal in most dis-eases). Consider the preponderance of sexual dysfunction and incontinency. Consider how overrun by pharmaceuticals our lives and bodies have become. We have become as reckless with our bodies as we have in our relationship to the bodies of the Earth.

Consider also man's inhumanity to man. We had to create the word "genocide"; people have continuously destroyed whole groups of other people because of their skin color, religious beliefs or cultural differences. We have hatred personified in genocide. (Genocide Convention 2002). Historically, it has existed probably since the beginning since nothing is new on the planet.

How can we be so compassionless and soul-less to do such things? Would we think to do this to another, if we remembered who we really were or where we really came from? We just keep replaying the same old stupid stuff over and over again…and we will continue to do this until we realize we are killing ourselves, as we thoughtlessly kill each other and this beautiful planet.

Now, consider the conditioned thought-feelings we carry with us that we project onto others: ie. "I'm not enough and neither is anyone else", "I feel so wrong that I have to overcompensate and be right about everything, making everyone else wrong, so I can pretend to feel safe and loved", self righteousness, self importance, self criticism, self rejection, self loathing, etc., etc., etc. These programs create bedlam for us.

We do not fare well in relationships—of all kinds—because: 1) we have not learned to be responsible for our creations, 2) we do not know what to do when we are confronted by our creations, so we deny and avoid them, 3) we constantly blame, judge and make wrong others and then pretend to be happy. 4) Mostly, we just run away and hide in substances, people or schedules.

Most of us live dissonant lives. Our habits of living prove our disconnect to God, to the Earth, to our bodies and to each other. How we live and who we have become exist because we flounder outside our true nature—our true essence.

Most of us do not remember Origin; we do not remember how Creation came into being. As a result, we have no real foundation for our existence. Not knowing our original birth, our Original Parents and the circumstances of our birth disempowers us.

As a consequence we are left very much to our own devices. We are left with an individuated mind that believes it knows everything. It does not. What it knows is Separation...and the controlling ego within that mind does its utmost to maintain that position much to our detriment. (Ceanne DeRohan, Right Use of Will, Original Cause, etc. and A Course in Miracles)

What else are we left with? We are left with the absolute beauty of our precious bodies—our Earthly bodies—the physical, emotional, mental and spiritual bodies which were given to us as schools of learning. **OUR BODIES KNOW EVERYTHING.** They remember where we come from. They know we are infinitely connected to the Body-Mind of God-Goddess. Our bodies have a wisdom that keeps us honest in the middle of our conditioned dishonesty.

The nature of our bodies is to get us to reconnect with God-Goddess, with the Earth (of which we are a significant part), with ourselves and with each other. The nature of our bodies is to get us to realize that we are Eternal and that we can remember and indeed reclaim the Life Abundant...Life Everlasting. We can also reclaim rememberance and observance of the Universal Truths that Diversity is Our Natural State and that We are All One.

It is my belief that all of humanty is headed into Union with Source; that our bodies are already undergoing a purification (as is the Earth) and an accelerated evolutionary process that is indeed changing our physiology. As we awaken to this wondrous process, we can align with it and make our part and the part of the whole less traumatic and more graceful.

Don't look to science for your answers. Don't look to religion. (What religion is God anyway?). Don't look to any form of government as your authority. These institutions are not a part of your nature. They were created through abuse. Abuse of the path of power created religion. Abuse of the path of service created politics. Abuse of the path of mind created science.

Look within to find Divine Wisdom, Divine Intelligence, Divine Trust, Divine Knowing, Divine Freedom. Look within to find the answers to all your questions...God is your Science, your Religion, your Government. Living with God as your co-pilot is your true nature.

Seek to know God, don't just learn about God. Follow God, not church leaders. (Anna Lee Skarin, Beyond Mortal Boundaries.)

I did not know all of this in the beginning, I did not remember God, nor my connection, so I bought into the conditioning I was born into. Now that I know better, I know I can question everything. And now that I have reclaimed my feeling nature, I know what is real and what is possible. Anna Lee Skarin says, "It is impossible for one to keep going and not get there."

And…to tell my story, we must start from the beginning when I did not know.

2) CHILDHOOD

I knew about death and dying at a young age. No, it was not vicariously through a relative passing. It was my own personal experiences. I learned about it from the nuns and priests when I was in 3rd grade at St. Augustine's Catholic parochial school in Bayview, Wisconsin. The teachings, pictures and sermons on hell and damnation grabbed me by the throat. This information, in my mind, translated into "Be obedient-do it right or your punishment will be death".

I was such an empath, that I managed to soak up all the fear and terror of my classmates as well as my own. Consequently, I looked forward to daily Mass with much dread and trepidation. I became so nervous about the whole thing that my parents and family doctor put me on tranquilizers at the tender age of eight.

Shortly thereafter, I started having very sharp pains in my heart. I knew I was dying for sure then. It is amazing how inventive and dramatic we are with our imaginations. I held on month to month like Veronica Lake on her deathbed. I posed the question often to myself: "I wonder if I will be here at Easter?" Then I would query about the next holiday—they were my markers.

I dared not tell anyone of my plight or fright. My parents were too busy feeding, clothing and raising five kids and a chihuahua. So, I just kept it to myself as I lay awake at night praying to Jesus to please let me see Christmas, etc.

Little did I know that being "high strung"(as I was told I was), rendered me very retentive in the fecal department. Who wouldn't be in a noisy household with a yelping "high strung" dog? (Curiously…she favored me). As a result, I learned to live in a very constipated state.

Thus, I felt continuously nauseous, pained in my colon and my heart and frazzled that I would soon be dead.

I remember people telling my parents when I was little (2 years of age or so), "My, your little girl is so serious". If they hardly ever defecated, they would have been serious too. Maybe this can support us in giving understanding to all those "Crabby Appletons" in our lives. But, I digress here.

When most young children are running around like little indians, carefree and happy with nary a concern in the world about them, there I was, taut with anxiety and dread, and grim about the immediate future...I felt obsessed by death and the process of dying.

(Curiously, it IS the colon where all physical death begins anyway. A dirty, sludged up colon will kill all the organs, putrify the fluids and exhaust the body into all kinds of dysfunction, degeneration and decay. Of course, the mind also is another major player in this process as well. With the average american lifestyle and it 's accompanying near unconsciousness, it takes about 75-80 years to kill a body).

I am not exactly sure what it was that took my focus off death as a child, but it very well could have been the night I believed that the Virgin Mary appeared to me. I was between ages 11 and 12. Sure...I could have imagined or dreamed it. All I know is that She appeared in the corner of my bedroom in a white, golden, blue radiance. She told me not to worry...that ALL WAS WELL and that I was going to be helping people.

After She left , I felt very relaxed in my body. I don't remember worrying about dying after that night. In retrospect it was probably the first Divine intervention this lifetime that I have consciousness of. It was shortly after that, that my Dad bought me my first hi-fi. I started listening to music, I began dancing and my mind turned to other things.

3) YOUNG ADULTHOOD

At the age of 27, I "awoke" one sleepless night to the realization that there was something terribly wrong with my marriage. My spouse could shed no light on the matter. For the next four years, we pretended to do life together, as we fell into rapid disrepair.

I, meantime, did everything I could to run away through activity. Within 3 years of suppressed emotional baggage, I created a bonafide case of rhuematoid arthritis. It felt like a death sentence to my young body-mind. "Isn't that the disease that cripples old people and don't they wind up in wheelchairs and nursing homes?" I shuddered.

I told the rhuematologist (the best in Milwaukee, Wisconsin) that I wanted to approach this condition as wholistically as possible. He said, "That's the only way I do it…here, take these pills". I said, "No, you don't understand". And he said,"NO, Miss, you don't understand. You will always have this disease and you have three choices. You can take these pills (Clinoril—an anti-inflammatory) two times a day or you can take 12-16 aspirin a day or you can live with the pain".

I reluctantly took the pills vowing silently to not take them. I lasted about 3 days; the pain was making me insane…it was so intense. It kept intensifying and the M.D.'s suggestion each time was "up your dosage of the medication". When I was taking twice the recommended pharmaceutical dose, I asked about side affects. He did not know…and suggested that I read the printout in the PDR. That was when I decided I really needed to become my own doctor.

I began investigating different options and started working with shifting my diet and taking alfalfa—the supposed grandfather of herbs. I started feeling better in a short time. I felt stronger. I asked the rheumatologist what he thought of taking alfalfa. He snorted and said,

"You want to know how many of my patients have tried alfalfa?" I thought to myself, " Yes, but how many have tried it and never come back to see you?".

I followed the rheumatologist's advice for two months and then took leave of his services. It felt to me like he was advocating for the dis-ease and himself more than he was advocating for me. I began reading everything I could get my hands on with regard to this dis-ease. I began to realize that many doctors and even the Arthritis Foundation did not work to support people out of this dis-ease.

"Intent is the art of healing with feeling", according to Dr. Ted Morter. Dr. Morter says that negative or indifferent intent impairs healing. He says that a doctor who intends nothing but improvement for his or her patient is practicing intentional healing; that intention is the common denominator in healing. It felt like the rheumatologist I had gone to, practiced negative intent in his terror tactics. Had I believed him, I would have never healed anything.

Rheumatoid arthritis is an equal opportunity employer—it gives every joint and muscle group a chance to experience trauma and pain. When you have a traumatized joint, the heat and pain of the area exceed the circumference of the area. It radiates well beyond the body…it renders a person almost senseless. It incapacitates us.

With continued dietary changes, alfalfa and a lifestyle change (I separated, then divorced my husband—I was heavy into blame at that time, because I did not know better). I went into remission for a year, visited the tryanny of pain for about two more years and then was free of it for a long time (until my senility years). Rebirthing, Massage, Reiki, Body Electronics and Quantum Dynamics moved the arthritis out of my body and kept it at bay for 16 years. I required no medication during that time because I had no pain or physical limitations.

Even though I got a reprieve in the physical pain department, I still had not thoroughly addressed the emotional pain. As a consequence, I continued to run away through activity. I "successfully" pulled this off for a number of years; working 90 plus hours a week—two full time jobs and a ton of priorities. Self importance is a game of running away through activity that can kill you.

I started changing my lifestyle in March of 1985 after I got a message from Ram Dass (Mahavatar Babaji of Hairakhan's Ram Dass). I had flown home from a National Convention for The American Massage Therapy Association where I had been involved in meetings (I was on the National Board and State President for Wisconsin) and workshops for 10 days.

I drove directly from the airport to my appointment with Ram Dass. He was touring the U.S., doing exquisite accupuncture healings. He did a session on me which may have been the 4 windows. It took me directly to Heaven within myself. It was an exceptional experience.

At the conclusion of the session, he told me that it was imperative that I change how I did my life. He said if I did not, that I would be dead in a short time. I heard him and recognized that this was God talking to me thru him. I took steps to change my life gradually and consistently. I had opportunity to change a lot.

I had a live in boyfriend move out. I stopped smoking cigarettes. I stopped drinking alcohol. I stopped doing recreational drugs. I cleaned up my lifestyle and started taking better care of myself.

Even though I made a bunch of changes, I was still overworking. I was enjoying what I was doing...I did a lot of spiritual practices and inner work, along with all my other priorities. I filled my time and I recognized that I was still burning the candle at both ends.

4) TIME FOR A CHANGE

It was probably in '87 or '88 that I started getting the message that I needed to leave Wisconsin or I would die. So I started praying to Mother Father God to take me where I needed to go…to do what it was that I needed to do. I had no idea what that would be.

I knew I would be leaving teaching in the public sector (I had been teaching High School Spanish and English for 19 years and I loved it), but I did not know I would be quitting massage (I had gone from doing psychotherapy to massage because I found it to be a bigger support in my and other people's lives). I did not know what I would be doing. I just knew it would be different.

I told myself I would be doing God's work, but the truth was that I was running away from an unhealthy relationship that I did not know how to quit and from an emotionally abusive, rebellious teenage son who had fired me as his mother. Nope, that is not the real truth. The real truth is that I was running away from myself.

I also did not know that this was the stage that I created to let me know that I was done in Wisconsin and that another reality was about to be created…another assignment…another school of learning. All I had to do is be willing to close the door on the past for the new door to open.

When Babaji told me to become a Quantum Dynamics Teacher, I was squeamish about it. I feared Jim Dvorak, the Master Q.D. Teacher (past life stuff), but I acquiesced. In June of 1990 I came to New Mexico for what I thought would be a 2 week training. Jim and Mary Byrne (Jim's partner and an exceptional Q.D. Teacher in her own right) compressed time. My process and spiritual evolution got greatly accelerated. I worked with them for 5 and a half months and I was nowhere near the same person. I was consciously fearless for the first time in memory.

The message was clear. I was to relocate to New Mexico. I went back and forth from Wisconsin to New Mexico six times between June and November, taking care of emptying my home and bidding farewell to my relations. In autumn of 1990 I chose Las Cruces to move to…or maybe it chose me.

The Organ Mountains are exceptional. Every time I drove past them on the way to the airport in El Paso, Texas these mountains seemed to be calling me. They have an extraordinary energy about them, but then so does Las Cruces, N.M. The first time we had pictures taken of the Earth from outer space, three lights or bright spots appeared on those photographs. Las Cruces was one of those lights.

In late November of that year, when I came to network with more New Mexicans, I met Dr. Kelley Elkins, a very non-traditional Dr. of Chiropractic. I had planned to stay for only a few weeks, but I never really went back to Wisconsin. God's plan was stronger than mine.

Kelley had prayed for a teacher for about six months. Then when I showed up, he fought me tooth and nail. (Amazing how we fall back on ourselves when the Universe starts fulfilling our desires). He was a very willing student, but a not so willing partner—which was not my idea. I kept surrendering to Babaji—He kept assuring me that this was my right place.

It took us a good year and a half to get through a bunch of our old conditioning, before we could truly appreciate the gifts and value we had together. Once we found this, our relationship became excellent and dynamic.

What Kelley and I created together was a partnership of trust, surrender and understanding—not between us, but within ourselves. We trusted ourselves in the presence of the other. We surrendered our conditioning, to be able to experience the truth of ourselves with each other.

We understood that what we were together, in God-Goddess' plan was bigger than both of us. These places we came to within ourselves, allowed us to overcome our pasts; to live in the present moment of now, to dedicate ourselves to loving God-Goddess, to healing our stuff and to committing to one another.

We eventually recognized the soul commitment of being together. It seems very clear that **WE ARE HERE TO HEAL RELATIONSHIP; OUR RELATIONSHIP TO MOTHER-FATHER GOD** and all aspects of self, to become whole and Holy once again. Once we heal these sacred relationships, healing issues with everybody else is a cinch, since all our relationships are just reflections of this primary sacred relationship.

We also recognized that we agreed to do this senility project together. If I had not left Wisconsin when I did (when I was directed to do so), I would not have met Kelley and he and I were to do this piece together. There is no doubt in my mind. Without him caretaking me and daily lifting me out of the sludge of senility, I would not have survived.

5) PRELUDE TO SENILITY AND EEP

I do not believe I was "awake" enough as a child, adolescent or young adult to recognize my empathic nature and what that meant for my health and well being. I remember one of my high school students sharing with me that his Dad had married a woman so sensitive that they could not live in the city because of the people energy. Little did I know that I would become that sensitive as well, as I became more conscious by emptying my old conditioned programs.

I had been Rebirthing for 5 years and worked with Body Electronics for about 3 years, when I got initiated into Quantum Dynamics in 1985. Q.D. as it is called, was a lifesaver for me. Q.D. is an amazing tool. It is so practical; it allows us to let go of upsets in 10 seconds or less. It also allows us to address thought and feeling and change it into energy and light. I love it.

Q.D. allowed me to drop my addictions and ill serving habits. It changed my life several times for the better. With it, I was able to let go of my white knuckle death grip on life (along with a lot of old conditioned terror, fear, and blaming anger, hatred and rage) and let go of my attachments to people, places and the past. In 1990 I became a Q.D. Teacher.

Between 1985 and the intensive training in 1990 I did with Jim Dvorak and Mary Bryne to become a Q.D. Teacher (which also involved a lot of Rebirthing and Spiritual Purification), I emptied so much of my psychological debris that my already empathic nature got greatly amplified. I could read and feel what other people were thinking and feeling—often I knew things about them that they had no clue about themselves. It was a great boon in supporting my clients in their process.

Equipped with the above mentioned tools, Massage (I was a Registered Massage Therapist) and Reiki (I was level II in the Usui tradition at the time), plus my own personal empowerment (as a result of being accelerated in my process from working with masterful teachers), I felt fearless and ready for whatever it was that God-Goddess wanted me to do next.

In 1990, when it became clear that I was to relocate to New Mexico (I had received about nine messages the previous 3 years that I would be living in the southwest), I surrendered to the Plan. When I met Kelley, I saw and felt how nicely his B.E.S.T. (Bio Energetic Synchronization Technique- a non-invasive, soft tissue manipulation) wedded with Q.D., breathwork and my other tools. It felt like a great match.

Our technologies together became the foundation…the pathwork for ourselves and our clients. Spiritual Purification (the ancient practice of working with the elements) also became an established practice for us, as well as many East Indian, Native American and Shamanistic rituals and ceremonies.

While I was fearless, strong and ready for just about anything when I met Kelley, I also had emptied so much of my programming, that my sensitivity pretty much disallowed me from spending large blocks of time with people who were not doing the same.

At that time I did not know Leonard Orr's (the Father of Rebirthing) term "emotional energy pollution", but I did know what it felt like to be grabbed up by people's unconscious death urge and programming. And, I knew when people and disembodied energies were near me or in me. I had learned to really feel.

Emotional Energy Pollution is the trail we leave of ourselves wherever we travel. It is like we are continuously unravelling ourselves. This energy, unbeknownst to us, is like a slime trail that interacts with everyone and everything we come into contact with. Our trail is our own denied, suppressed, repressed mental-emotional baggage. It contains death urge and conditioned patterns of behavior, thought and emotions-feelings. We exchange EEP with folks all day long when we live in the world.

Lyall Watson writes,"We are, it seems, electric animals with sensitive magnetic minds, caught up in a web of electro-magnetic influence. And it is somewhere in this energetic web that we have to look for the impetus that made us conscious and gave us the ability to knit ourselves into such an electropollution tangle". (p.103, <u>Gifts of Unknown Things</u>)

Becker in <u>The Body Electric</u> writes,"It may be a little disconcerting to know that we and all living things are surrounded by a magnetic field extending out into space from our bodies and that the fields of the brain reflect what is happening in the brain. The implications of this are enormous". (1990, p. 70)

In the beginning years of my heightened sensitivity (early '90s), I would cough and then sometimes gag with EEP. I could easily release this energy with a head turn (the Eagle's Breath) with Q.D. Sometimes, my vision would get blurry or I would get to feeling a bit dizzy or "off". As the years progressed, working with more people and attracting more folks who came without their bodies, this energy became denser in my bodies.

No doubt, my bodies were breaking down getting denser from the EEP. It now became painful. I am certain that a portion of this pain was my defense physiology—my defended reaction-response to what I was feeling, along with my judgement and fear of what I was feeling.

The "unwashed public" (people who have done no inner work) carry so much garbage. I must say that many healers themselves feel pretty bad as they take on other people's EEP and do not continuously move it. Leonard Orr himself has said that sometimes it is easier to be around ordinary folks, because Rebirthers tend to have their stuff hanging all around them. This has been my experience with many Reiki Masters, psychics and channels I have met as well.

Leonard maintains that the highest service is to process other people's stuff. He also says that processing other people's stuff produces a net gain for the person doing it. So, being the beneficiary of a psychic attack can have its rewards. I have experienced the latter many times, but I do not agree with Leonard's first premise. The reason I don't is because I feel it is a disservice to take karmic opportunity away and to take that on.

AND I know that EEP can kill and I am not willing to die for anybody. But then Leonard isn't willing to die for anyone either. He says Jesus tried that and it didn't work. Are you aware that it didn't work? Jesus didn't die for your sins, but you may die from the conditioning you have in your body around what you have been taught are "sins" you believe you have committed…IF you don't wake up and do something about it NOW and continuously!

I believe our opportunity is to learn self preserving and healthful new definitions for LOVE, compassion, sympathy, empathy and pity. Too often, Christianity in this country believes that all of these terms fall under the category of love. They absolutely do not.

The Science of Compassion can teach us a lot if we are willing to let go of everything we have learned, believed and been indoctrinated into thinking and doing as habit. We do not empower ourselves or others by fishing for them. We cannot save others from themselves, but we can direct them into seeing the folly of their miscreations and their conditioning.

The Science of Compassion is about tough love and absolute loving detachment from everyone and everything. Christ did not fall into a person's "poor me"" case; if he had, there would have been two people in need of help. And, he did not acknowledge every person's presence or request. He knew how to feel and he knew who was genuine and ready to accept the responsibility of a healing.

I thought I was handling the EEP. I bathed two—three times a day, daily I did Q.D. process or Rebirth or both, daily I got B.E.S.T. work done on me, daily I smudged. I thought I was following my highest desire. I was conscientious with my diet—I played on and off with being a vegetarian and drank only pure water. I did fire often (had candles going 24-7 in the house, did open fires outside several times a week, for a year I slept with fire nightly), did Sweat Lodge and Body Electronics often. I also did Reiki on myself daily and had others do full sessions on me. The EEP got me anyway.

EEP can get anyone, even God…when God is in body. It was EEP that took Babaji of Herakhan's body in February of 1984. It literally wore him out. He actually transitioned into Mahasamadi, left and recreated other bodies which are not readily available to the public at this time. Our own bodies contain so much toxicity that many immortals choose to not be around us, but Babaji was willing to do this for us.

When you consider it, it was EEP that took all the great healers: Edgar Cayce, Phineas Quimby, John Christopher, Katherine Kohlman. My friend, Jim Self, founder of Avalon Institute in Chico California and an excellent healer in his own right, said that Katherine died of everything. She had every dis-ease in her body: every dis-ease she supported people in releasing from their body went into her—she did not know how to release it. Jim said she did not know how to ground herself or create her own healing space apart from those she worked with. None of these healers knew how.

It also took me a while to recognize that the Higher Purpose I had identified for myself was killing me: "Do whatever it takes to heal The Mother of Everything within myself and everyone who is willing to do the work…even if it means dying to accomplish this goal". I did not uncover this last bit, until I was well into senility. I did not see my old conditioning until it was well into my body. Death is a sad choice for people to take to get to Heaven. They won't find heaven outside of themselves.

6) THE LOSS OF POWER

November 19th, 1997 we retired late after midnight. We were exhausted, having had a full day of work, then packing, getting ready to get up early to head north to Albuquerque and then Santa Fe. We had clients in both locations and would be gone a week to ten days.

After about an hour, I awoke as I lay on my left side, to a very loudly, pounding erratic heartbeat. I quickly turned over to my back only to feel it intensify. It terrified me. It felt like it was galloping and was outside of my body.

Usually, I would wake Kelley to have him ask Divine Intelligence through my feet (like dowsing) what was going on. But he was really crabby and exhausted when he retired, so I did not disturb him. It was probably a very poor decision on my part. In the long run, it cost me a lot.

Instead, I lay there in terror, breathing, processing 4th Chakra stuff with Q.D. which probably saved my life. I was awake all night. I did manage to get my heart to settle down a bit, but it continued to worry me. Over the next several months, my heart continued to beat erratically on occasion and my health deteriorated. It was as if my confidence in the stamina and strength of my body went down the tubes.

The ensuing year ('98), I went in and out of good health and well-being. We had not taken a vacation nor had down time is six years. In March, I got the message very loudly that we needed to get away even for a short time. So we planned a five day get away. It was great, but felt not enough…so that year we took many vacations. I thought, "If I just take time off, away from work, I will regene myself…especially as I continue to work my process".

My legs, knees and feet got more and more achey…and then they would be ok. I went back and forth. I felt ok and then I would feel lousy. My own mind plagued me with doubt about my health.

In December of 1998, during a workshop in Santa Fe, one of our clients showed us some products from Dr. Richard Schulze. We did not even have to read about it. We felt the life force and opportunity with these products. We began taking them immediately.

Even though Dr. Schulze's products were great, the die had been cast. When we went for our last working vacation to Big Sur, in January of 1999, my body was struggling to maintain. I was getting slower in my gait and I hurt. My fear was accelerating.

I did Dr. Schulze's 30 Day Incurables Program and felt great after I did my first cold sheet treatment. Two days later I could not move. Apparently, I pulled out the cork to the repressed material my body had been holding. When it began its journey outward, I was devastated.

By the end of March, I could not get up and walk to the bathroom or stand alone in the shower. I was writhing in pain and experiencing more and more symptomatology each day. I counted more than 50 symptoms at one point. Kelley could hardly touch me to work on me; he was beside himself not knowing what to do. Sometimes I just cried and screamed with the unabating pain.

By late summer, early fall, I felt totally victimized by other people's energies and I felt trapped in a body that did not work for me. My parents who were in their late seventies and in failing health, were continuously coming into my body; I was feeling the dysfunction within their bodies…and they were thousands of miles away.

I learned later that the episode with my heart was not even me. It was my father who was in sympathy with my brother. My brother had had a quintriple bypass two years previously. AND…my brother's heart episode was not him; he was doing it for his lover. Not only are we One Mind, we are One Body.

In the debilitated state I was in, I seemed to magnetize more and more of other people's energy. My own fear, terror and dread was exacerbated by the presence of these energies. I also had some clients who I was so emotionally enmeshed with, that I could not get free of their energy. I felt in continual struggle. I felt like I was holding the EEP of the Planet and I was loathesome to it.

I was confused about what was going on with me. I said to myself that I did not know what was happening. I guess fear masked the denial. I wanted to say "it" took me by surprise, but as stated it was a gradual process of degeneration, accumulation of death urge and EEP. So many different theories flooded my consciousness and information was given to Kelley and me piecemeal.

7) OH MY GOD…IT'S SENILITY

Kelley was the first to recognize it for what it was: SENILITY. It seems out of a fog I remember him calling it senility and telling me just to accept it…that I would get thru it. Recalling this now is like listening to a voice in a dream in a faraway tunnel. I did not hear it at first…so great was my denial. It was kind of like the numb terror I went into when that rheumatologist told me I had rheumatoid arthritis at age 32.

It's that place of dread that we experience in the face of something that we just "know" from our conditioning is going to be "unsurvivable" and "undo-able". I am certain it is the kind of terror and panic—like no exit terror that prompts people into killing themselves, rather than facing and going into the dreaded experience whatever it is. Some people choose death over fear. All I know is that senility and all that that could mean scared the crap out of me.

When the reality of the situation started settling in, I felt completely at no choice. I was in dramatic overload, can't hide, hopelessness and devastation. It was a totally horrific and frightening experience to watch my body-mind literally decay in front of my very eyes.

Leonard Orr, the father of Rebirthing, is the first senility graduate I know. He has championed eight terminal dis-eases…he did that in a five year period. He is still dealing with the residual physical stuff and recovering from the financial devastation, while rebuilding his career and Rebirthing around the world.

Leonard is the only person I know to write about senility as a passage to Physical Immortality. His contributions in this realm are invaluable. People need to wake up around this. While we have plenty of time, time is of the essence. We must be taking action or we will not reap the Glory that is ours. Leonard has many publications on this topic. His book <u>Breaking the Death Habit</u> is superlative and a must read for this research. (You can order it from him at Rebirth International/Inspiration University, P.O. Box 1026, Staunton, VA. 24402. 540-885-0551).

Senility is an altered state of consciousness where all past trauma and issues from life surface spontaneously and simultaneously. Everything that has not been handled (processed into light) from intra-uterine memory through infancy, childhood, adolescence, and adulthood come crashing into your body-mind at the same time.

Every dis-ease that has been created through the thought forms and emotional conditioning you have taken on from your family—your geneology, from your own programs or karma, from your death urge and from the accumulated EEP and death urge of other people, birth themselves in your body at the same time in senility.

It is a state of intense feelings and overwhelm. I felt completely and totally engulfed in victim consciousness; I felt hopeless, depressed, suicidal. I felt like death urge was oozing out of every cell of my being. As a result, I felt incredible dread, fear, terror—no exit terror. No exit terror is feeling like you are supremely trapped and there is no place to turn to and no place to hide.

Struggle to maintain consciousness for even a minute, to remember to breathe was a constant. Even though I was a practicing Rebirther for 19 years prior to this, I could not maintain a connected breath…forget about a breath release. I could not remember to stay on purpose. It was like I kept falling into holes in my brain. I could not maintain continuity of thought, breath or action. My speech was also dramatically affected.

I could not pull myself out of it. I could not even do an Eagle's Breath (Q.D. release). I felt like I was continually fragmenting…and then regrouping with less and less of myself each time. It was like the death urge had me by the throat doing the tango and it was leading. I could not follow, but it did not care and would not let go of me. There was no escaping from it.

The pain I experienced took me to new depths of despair. It seemed that nothing could alleviate the torture. I only took aspirin and frequently that did not help. I screamed, I cried. I took pity on myself and my situation. Not being able to function, I felt locked in "can't".

I found it impossible to sleep at night because of the pain and discomfort. Short naps of fifteen minutes was all my body would allow me during the day. I went almost the whole first year without sleep, being constantly exhausted.

As a consequence,I was whiney and crabby. I just wanted to"wah" my head off and I did not care who heard or what they thought . (Of course there was no one around but Kelley, God bless him). I prayed a lot and found little comfort in prayer or God.

I really felt like a failure…a total failure. My personal lie of "not enough" was up major big time. I felt entombed in infancy consciousness….except I could not even crawl. I felt at no choice, hopeless, helpless and ashamed of not being able to pull myself out of this state.

This body-mind state really frightened me. Formerly, I had believed there was no condition that I, or anyone else, created that we could not uncreate. After all, I had pulled myself out of crippling rheumatoid arthritis. If I had done that, then surely I could do it again.

But nothing seemed to work on me. It was like my body was dead already. It was so unresponsive to any therapy we did. B.E.S.T. chiropractic, Quantum Dynamics, traditional chiropractic (Thompson technique), Reiki, Body Electronics, massage. Everything that had always worked brilliantly on me before, seemed totally ineffective now.

It was like the self-destruct mechanism was on full tilt and there was nothing to do, but watch my body die. Suicide became a frequent visitor on my intermittent brain waves. It would present itself and then somehow my life force would rise to my consciousness and overtake the darkness.

I was very youthful looking before I began this lela. At 50, I looked 10 years younger. One year into this, I started aging rapidly. Dr. Schulze, herbalist par excellance of American Botanical, talks about women going thru endocrine and immune dysfunction dis-eases. They are so adversely affected that he says they look like they age 150 years. I know exactly what he is talking about.

I've also heard that complaining, ages us. I did not care...I had never been so awfully miserable in my life and I felt betrayed by my body. My hands became incredibly arthritic looking and feeling. I was able to use my hands and arms less and less. My knees, ankles and feet were swollen. The big toe on the left foot and the toe next to it, began moving as a bunion birthed itself and the bones of the feet moved, so that none of my boots or shoes fit me, except my birkenstocks.

My muscles atrophied quickly from misuse. (Apparently, atrophy starts setting in after as little as 24 hours). At first they got very soft, then they turned into pudding and then they seemed to disappear altogether. My skin lost its tonicity and became very dry and wrinkly. In places on my legs, my skin appeared shiny. I lost a tremendous amount of weight...and I was only about 110 lbs. to begin with.

Sometimes I could walk. Sometimes Kel would have to carry me. I could not get up and down from the sofas or our futon bed. The first six months, I slept on my massage table, because it was easier for Kel to work on me. Kelley then built us a beautiful tall bed.

I had so many things going on with me...so many symptoms. I felt chronically ill. I just felt sick, yucky and green. I was either freezing or bathed in sweat both winter and summer. My body odor was foul. It smelled like the bodies of folks in old people's homes or like the death of hospitals.

I felt aged and I looked aged. I walked like a little old lady—all bent up, shuffling around...when I could walk. I frequently staggered, bumped into walls and things. I often felt like I was losing my balance. I actually went through several weeks off and on of vertigo. I dropped food all over myself and my peeing aim was poor, much to the chagrin of my spouse.

I felt decrepid and dried up. I was losing my body, my mind, muscle strength, personal strength…my personal power. My sentiency and empathic abilities were destroyed by the pain and continuous trauma. My body-mind shut down so badly that I vacillated between pain and numb…I felt little else.

I was falling into an incredibly huge black hole. It was a heavy, dark space that was at times scorchingly dry, and at other times uncomfortably moist and sticky. I felt maxed out in motionlessness, breathlessness…as if I was caught in a time warp. I felt like I was in hell. Everything was blurry or off kilter. Nothing was concrete or abstract. It felt like insanity.

I was in an abyss of poor me, struggle, suffering and abject poverty. I felt like an invalid, painted on a canvas by another's brush. I was trapped. I could only breathe fear and a sickening heaviness in and out. I felt lost in a nightmare.

I could not read or write most of the time because my eyes and mind did not work. I did manage a few journal entries here and there. There were also a few times that I could feel normal enough to process myself or another, and then I would crash back into the senility pattern.

8) IN THE SPIRAL OF DARKNESS

The following are some verses that speak to the body-mind space that I occupied in the throes of Senility. They were written about two years later in memory of the state that I championed.

IN THE MIDDLE OF IT

Darkness played everywhere
    like a heavy mantle, inside
        and outside of my eyelids…
        threatening to suffocate me.
    It was insufferably patient.

Wide eyed, caught in a web
        of tyranny,
    I waited to be devoured.

Endure……I must! Breathe!!!
Life's temptation……to expire.

How rude and cruel the wait.
How loud and long the silence.
How ungodly my existence……

PAIN

Christ! Stop! Your nails do penetrate me too much!
Deep within my fabric do the spasms consume me.
Intolerable fire and piercing rage does my body shriek.
Wrest your grip from me you dishonorable horror.
                    Let me be......Just let me be.

HUSHED

My body-mind became a muted instrument.
It offered no song; but creaked from misuse.
    My hands no longer saw;
        my eyes no longer caressed...
            what was once their passion.
Betrayed was I, like a minstrel with no audience.
Silent to the world, as the spittel ran down
            the side of my unsuspecting face.

HOLY WATER

Sweat poured forth from every fiber
            of my being.
A heat so intense, it likely fried
            my brain.
I wondered how faired my innards
    as I lay saturated in a puddle of
            newly expressed liquid.
Agni, my friend, lit me up hourly
    to purify me from the inside out.

Sister, my sister, do not fret about
    your little summer.
Sister, my sister, do not imagine that
    your holy water is not blessed.
Sister, my sister, your body is a sacred vessel,
    purifying humanity from the scourge
        of their repressed rage.
Sister, my sister, Heart of the Earth, bleed forth your sweat
    from the sanctity of your soul......
        that you may be freed as well.

ALONE

Betrayed by my body,
    I lay frozen in time.
My mind trapped in an endless tunnel
    of hollow despair.
Numb holes did fill me
    with an eternity of broken promises.
God, where were you?

Throughout this period, Kel worked on me constantly. I would do water, do fire, feel better; feel bad, read some Leonard, feel better; feel yucky, get worked on, feel better. I could not maintain the good space for very long—minutes to hours—then back to the muck of senility.

(The above partial poem and paragraph are remnants of a larger piece of writing that got corrupted on my C drive as I was finishing the book. When I went to see if I could recall the energy of that time frame, my body-mind would not do it. What I had written is not a loss, because what I have now is a return to aliveness and health that I am eternally grateful for.)

9) POVERTY IS A DIS-EASE

We had no idea how long this process would take. It took far longer than we wanted it to. Senility is a full time job for the caretaker and the person doing it. In a very real sense, we both were doing it, because it engulfed both of us. It consumed every ounce of energy we had emotionally, physically, mentally, spiritually. It used us up good.

Financially it was devastating for us. We used up all of our savings at the end of the first year and then lived for a long while on plastic. Not only did I worry about my health, I really worried about how in the world we were going to pay our bills from month to month. We had fallen so far behind. Poverty consciousness and senility go hand in hand.

When I said earlier that senility is the stage where all unaddressed layers of your process come up at once, I meant it. There is no escaping it; it rises to the forefront of your theatre to make sure you do not miss it this time.

So…lack of money became as big an issue as all the dis-eases. Poverty consciousness truly is a dis-ease and truly is not the truth of who we are. Yet being as debilitated and degenerated as I became, I had a difficult time staying above the fear of the Collective that I seemed to be magnetizing faster to me than I could burn off and set free.

Poverty, like any dis-ease is a healing waiting to happen…You have to acknowledge and identify it, so you know what part of you is trying to get your attention. "What is the matter"? The matter is the thought forms, habits of belief, feelings, emotions, decisions, judgements you hold that have created this particular condition-situation-dis-ease.

Once you identify what "the matter" is, you get to realize that all that you hold around this dis-ease is what you agreed to carry in this lifetime or what you agreed to take on and that you agreed to heal it. And that what it is, says, reflects is not even the truth of who you are. AND…you did agree to bring it in, take it on and heal it, or it would not be a part of your experience.

10) LETTING GO

After a time, I had to surrender. Fighting it did not work. There was no way I could deny what was happening and resisting it only exacerbated everything. I finally got to a place where I could be the observer of my process in loving detachment. Mostly, I surrendered to doing it and learning from it.

For possibly the first time in my adult life I depended on another human being for my every movement and nearly every function. Before I met Kelley and before senility, I was very active, self sufficient and independent. I prided myself on my autonomy. I was always the caregiver; I was always directing the show.

Amazing how we play it safe, always being the one to give; there is very little responsibility involved. It feels like such a big responsibility to receive. We don't know how to be gracious about it. It almost feels embarrassing at first. It is also easier to pretend to be in control of our lives, when we are only participating with half of the Circle of Life. We appear to have less self worth than those we laud with our time, gifts, etc.

Many healers I know fall in this category…giving continuously, taking not for themselves, wearing themselves thin into the ground. Actually all beings have opportunity to: 1) better caretake themselves and 2) continuously allow themselves to find balance in giving and receiving.

Learning to receive is a humbling experience. It helps us be more compassionate and loving with ourselves. It also helps us let go of control and be better human beings. Reminder: Unconditional love comes from within us and pours out, not vice versa.

With Kelley's love and support and Babaji's (of Hairakhan is one of my connections to Source) constancy, I finally got to places where I could carve a niche on the mountain I was climbing and maintain a foothold. There were several of these markers, each of them provided a toehold and hope.

When I first became ill, we thought, "Oh, it is just another psychic attack". There was a woman in town who was not a nice lady…she was a "bad witch". Over the years, she manipulated people to use their energy and if she in anyway felt threatened by folks (power relationship), she would debilitate them and their energy. She had tried to take me out a few times before. But after we addressed her intervention, I did not improve.

At the end of the first year of decrepidness, we flew to meet with B.C. (British Columbia) Baba and Durga to see if they could help me. Durga got that I had been abducted by aliens or somebody and had been electrocuted to blow out my circuits, so I would not remember what they did to me. (Hey, in this business, no explanation is too outrageous for me). I immediately began releasing around it—electrocution—using Q.D. and for the first time in 9 months (or more), I could feel my legs and arms.

My mind also started to clear up. I perked up a bit, but I was still despondent and I looked pretty bad. I was skeletal, gaunt and greenish. People would tell Kelley how bad I looked. Their looks of fright told me. Being the catalyst for people to face their own mortality is not fun.

In March of 2000, my body-mind cleared even more when Babaji gave Kel and I the Bursting the Body Light-Violet Flame Forgiveness. We asked Babaji if He could teach us how to expand our Light Bodies in a quick and efficient way. The two breath meditations that are the BBL-VFF gave me the first big boost into healing the senility. It was yet another Divine intervention. I finally felt like I could now survive. I got my confidence back…thank you Mahavatar Babaji!

As I worked with the Bursting the Body Light-Violet Flame of Forgiveness breath meditations daily, my body-mind started waking up more and more. I started feeling myself and my sentiency began returning. I could now process myself with Quantum Dynamics and achieve a breath release with Rebirthing/Conscious Energy Breathing. I was happy.

I still needed aspirin. Without it, the pain was oppressive. I had a hard time thinking straight. Leonard encouraged me to go at least one day a week without aspirin, so I could process the pain. I did this for several months and then Leonard and Isabelle came to see me. They had just returned from another very successful treatment for Leonard for cancer at the Hoxey Clinic in Tiajuana, Mexico (Centro Bio-medico as it is called there). He was happy because he could feel the cancer leaving and he knew it was for good. He was healing the remnants of his senility.

Leonard brought me some Earth Magic, chinese herbs especially for arthritis sufferers. He had gotten these from Hoxey along with a book written by Richard Anderson—and his experiences with the same herbs. After 2 doses—6 tablets, I was able to walk both the left and right hand labyrinths on our property. I had not been able to walk them for two years. I was so happy! My knees were not thick, heavy and congested. I could move easily! It was a miracle. Thank you Goddess and thank you Leonard.

I did not maintain at that level, but I was much improved. My body could start to relax more without so much pain…I could finally catch up a bit. Without continuous distress, I was not so defended. I had a lot of catching up and a tremendous amount of healing to do. I still felt very debilitated and aged from two years of being ravaged from the effects of senility.

About a year and a half after taking the Earth Magic, I got to a place where it became ineffective. I got bummed, but Leonard helped turn that around. He said all that meant is that my body had experienced a "permanent significant gain". So now I periodically change off with the arthritis herbs and antioxidant supplements that I am taking, so I can have more permanent significant gains.

Letting go is learning to surrender. When we let go, we gain energy. When we hold back, we lose energy. Most of us withhold energy because we think that that is what keeps us safe as we continue to live in survival. And we all live in survival. We live as though we must defend ourselves continually against the onslaught of modern living and all of its "dangers". It is almost as though we are stuck in fight or flight without recognition of what we are doing...daily.

Survival in old conditioning translates to "barely making it; constantly struggling". This is a horrible way to perceive life and a miserable way to do it. This approach to life is very unloving. And whether we are conscious of it or not, this is the situation of the emotional body in all of humanity...actually in all of God's creatures on Earth. Thank Goddess we can release this habit and change it. We are all connected; as each and every one of us elects to let go, it affects the whole of the Earth.

Survival instead can be "loving the self enough to keep it from harm". Of course implicit in this decision is the need to know exactly what it is that we do to ourselves that is harmful...what habits, thoughts, beliefs, actions, words, feelings do we participate with often (if not daily) that cause us harm?

Surrendering is not giving up. It is giving in to your will. Your will is not separate from the Will of God. Your will is your emotional body and has a lot of healing to do. It is imperative that you awaken to your will in the process of surrendering to your life process and to all that your body has to teach you.

11) THE FALL

It was a not until January, 2001 that I actually saw the glimmer of light at the end of the tunnel. That was the day I fell and broke my left hip. I remember it well. Kel dropped me off in front of Walmart. I hobbled around like a little old lady. I felt fragile, elderly and weak. I hated the idea of living on plastic. As I went in to sign the receipt, it felt like our life and situation was pathetic.

I entered the check out lane behind Kel. He did not know I was there and he stepped back. I tottered. My right birkenstock (shoe) got caught on my left shoe. I went crashing down hard on my left side on concrete. I shrieked in horror, screaming out Kelley's name…feeling numb and terrified at the same time.

I started doing a connected breath immediately to compose myself, while Kel held me, doing Reiki on my head (he said I hit it pretty hard) and kept people away. I was in shock as I turned from my side to my back. Within about 10 minutes, I asked Kel to help me up. He lifted me over to a counter, where I realized that my left foot did not connect to my shoe or my body. (It was a most weird feeling!). I knew something was very wrong.

There was so much grace that day and so many gifts. We were on our way to our traditional chiropractor's office, so getting an x-ray was easy. On the way over, I called on every name of God that I knew and opened an Emergency MAP session with my MAP team that I had only started working with four days before. (Thank you Leonid Soboleff for sending me the book MAP: The Co-Creative White Brotherhood Medical Assistance Program).

I nearly allowed Kelley and our chiropractor, Ron Mitchell to talk me into going into the hospital. I managed, however, to maintain my own authorityship. Who was I kidding? I was already so compromised. If I had gone in to have a pin put into my hip, the hospital authorities would not have released me. They would have found all kinds of things "wrong" with me.

When doctors tell you what is "wrong" with you in their diagnosis, they are only guessing most of the time. Their guess can create far more harm than what is already going on. And, I wanted to work with my body in my own way. I did not want any complications—no side effects from misprescribed drugs and especially, I did not want to be opened up to staph infection, etc. I trusted the Divine Intelligence of my body to tell me what was going on. This is what I chose to continue to do.

Kel was willing to support me in my decision and I could tell he was fearful, never having attended to a femur-trochanter head break before. He relaxed after I reminded him what two mentors of ours had done.

Dr. Ted Morter, innovator of B.E.S.T. Chiropractic had a car crash into the left side of his car, forcing the femur head thru the acetabulum. Ted had his family doing B.E.S.T. chiropractic all day long, every day and was walking months before the surgeon who wanted to operate on him said he would be walking. (He was walking in two months compared to eight or nine).

Dr. John Ray, innovator of Body Electronics and other remarkable material, was working hard, burning the candle at both ends teaching his dynamic workshops. He fell asleep at the wheel late one night and crashed into a tree, caving in his rib cage on the steering wheel of his car. After the hospital called to notify his wife, she and a bunch of their friends kidnapped John from the hospital, took him home and plugged into him with their energy and the process of Body Electronics. They stayed plugged in til his ribcage came back up hours later…with no anesthesia!

Aren't our bodies incredible? We cannot come to know this unless we bother to take the time to find out what our bodies are capable of doing and then we must trust their regenerative ability. Why do people fear their bodies so?

By the time we got home, both Kel and I felt hopeful. As we pulled up, a neighbor was pulling out and helped Kel carry me into the house on a chair. Within minutes of our arrival, Norwood Yamini, a dear friend who is also the other non-traditional chiropractor in town arrived. He and Kel lifted me onto the massage table, which became my residence for the next three months.

That evening, eight hours after I fell, I had six members of my Spiritual Family plugged into me using Body Electronics. Two of them drove two and a half hours to get here. They helped me move old conditioned fear, anger, rage and stuckness that had been lodged in my pelvis. We transmuted it into incredible gratitude and celebration. There was so much love, giving and receiving at that table on my behalf. It was like God-Goddess were saying to me, "Now, tell us you're unsupported". I couldn't , because that was not the truth.

It became immediately clear in that session, that I had requested a "break" from the tyranny of senility, agedness, all the dis-eases and dysfunction in my experience. That's what I prayed for and that's what I got. As a result of that day, I have endeavored to be much more conscious in my languaging. I also owned how wrong I had made myself, senility, my body and what it was doing. I started releasing all of this and it started releasing me.

Except for a couple of moments of old conditioned fear, I was high on this opportunity. It seemed like this was the closing of the door of what had been (in terms of conditioning) and a new portal had opened up. I felt happy.

We enrolled Lucy Aristizabal, a sister in spirit and client to stay with us during my recuperation with the hip. Lucy had met Kel at a Rebirther's Convention in Virginia in 1995. As a result of a few minutes of conversation with him, she decided to come to New Mexico to work with us. She came for a week, stayed for a month and relocated here from New Jersey the following year.

It was a gift—the three of us being together at that particular time and space. We all needed the emotional and physical support. It was a tremendous give and take and healing that we did together. We all felt supported. We processed often, breathed Lucy, Luz and I got worked on often with B.E.S.T. from Kel. We toned often. We ate well, thanks to Kel's great culinary and baking skills that I had supported him in acquiring the previous year. Luz helped us financially for a few months and we helped her in an energetic transition within herself.

While Kelley had been my cheerleader from the beginning of this lela (God's play and learning), by mid 2000, he was burning out quickly. Not only was he doing everything for me and himself, he was also working like a mad man to get a website together for the Bursting The Body Light-Violet Flame of Forgiveness breath meditation and for A Next Step…light center for emotional healing. He did not know computers or the language. He was nearly as depressed as me the second half of 2000.

It is almost like when I fell, something broke in Kel too. It took him out of his hardness and despair. He was renewed again. It helped both of us so much to have Lucy present supporting us. I was and am still so grateful.

Most all my vanity and shame of body was taken away by all of this. You have to get over silly nonsense like that when you are dependent on others to change your diapers several times a day and several times at night and sponge bathe you. God bless them for loving me enough to do this for me. And God bless me for having the worthiness to have such a loving reflection.

Wearing diapers for 4 and 1/2 months was not the worst of my experiences. Lucy asked me one day if the infancy consciousness had increased from having to wear diapers. I had a lot of reservation in the beginning of having to be so dependent on others for particularly this function and I was able to overcome it quickly with their loving care. It was after all, just a fact of life…it was the "is-ness" of our lives at that point. We three met the challenge well.

The biggest discomfort was the heat. The plastic of the diaper prevented proper ventilation, so I was sweaty and uncomfortable. The biggest comforts were not having to worry about the pain of getting up to go to the bathroom. I could just pee and defecate and have it handled by two loving, honoring people. The other comfort was knowing that this was temporary. I was not incontinent. (By the way, I had some of the most incredible eliminations of my life after I fractured the hip).

While major fear producing symptoms seemed to end with the fracture, I still had fear to process out and it presented itself in a few different ways. I was up on crutches five weeks after I fell. I was not up well on them, but I was up. Probably two or three weeks after I began using the crutches to go to the bathroom, I was coming out of the bathroom by myself and I felt some urine run down my leg. It was most disconcerting, particularly because I had not felt any urge from my bladder. This continued to happen and I did get scared.

When we questioned Higher Intelligence, we found out that the bladder had been damaged in the fall. My fear sent me back into feelings of hopelessness and senility and infancy consciousness. I started processing around first chakra issues and potty training experiences. I also took steps to heal my bladder and kidneys with Dr. Schulze's kidney-bladder tea and his K-B flush. Within two weeks, I healed my bladder. I was grateful once again to Dr. Schulze.

Lucy introduced me to Dr. Samuel West's strategies working with a trampoline. Using a mini trampoline, you can create an electro-magnetic field of expanded consciousness with positive thought. Nearly everyday, Luz would jump on the trampoline while I toned names of God-Goddess and higher thought with regard to healing my body. It was awesome. I felt healthy and stronger than I had in a long time.

I also worked with my Map Team daily—sometimes more than once a day—on their suggestion. I believe they had a lot to do with my improved health as well. Whenever the pain got to be too much, I would call them in to advocate for me. Sometimes they would really alter my state with the work they did on my behalf.

I started exercising my arms and right leg. One of my friends told me that this would support all my body and the left leg from atrophying too much. Although admittedly, I was pretty atrophied at the time of the fall already from the previous years in senility.

During these first three months after the fall, Lucy and I read Harry Potter books—she for the first time and me for the second. Kel made homemade bread and cookies often as he had previously. Luz being with us made it into a bigger deal—more fun.

All of this helped raise my spirits. I was happier and healthier. It was probably not any one thing that created this state; it was the many gifts coming together. All of this contributed to raising my immune system. The fracture created the biggest boost to my immune system, I believe. I am not recommending it as a cure to anybody. I am just relating what I and Source created to bring me back to partial homeostasis.

Two months after the fracture, I fell again; this time, it was in my home and on my right side. I fell right in front of our altar in the living room. When Kel came home from a Co-op meeting in town and saw me there, he at first thought I was pranaming and praying. Then he realized that was not right…the way I was lying there. I felt foolish. I had taken too big a risk by myself. Even though it slowed my healing process, I got a net gain because I got to process a whole lot of fear of falling again.

12) BECOMING MY OWN DOCTOR

The rheumatologist in Milwaukee in 1979 was the last medical doctor that I went to. I figured, I had a better chance with me as the doc, since he seemed to be guessing anyhow. The more I learned about alternative health care and the miraculous results that people were receiving from Rebirthing, Colonics, Body Electronics, Reiki, Massage, Chiropractic, etc, the more I trusted the incredible gifts that lie within my body.

We are incredible beings. We have been given these magnificent holy temples to learn from. It is unfortunate that each time we incarnate, we return with such low consciousness and unknowing that we have to learn the hard way about what these physical bodies are about, what they are capable of and what they offer.

When God-Goddess put The Band Of Forgetfulness on us, we lost all memory of our grandness and what our lives were about millenia ago. We forgot that at one time we were so exquisitely connected and powered by Almighty God-Goddess that we held the same Divine Principles and Ways of Being that They embody. (What on Earth is Going On, 1997, Patricia Diane Cota-Robles, email: eraofpeace@aol.com; website: **www.1spirit.com/eraofpeace**).

We are on our way back to remembering, to creating Heaven on Earth in These Bodies Now, to living in Illumined Truth and Bliss, To Being Limitless, Physical Perfection and Freedom. AND…in order to do this, a person's individual lies and conditioning, must be found, acknowledged, transmuted and loved free from their earthly bodies.

No medical doctor or other human being or medical procedure can do that for us.

Acquiescing to the inevitability of death without questioning it is no way to live. It was never meant for us to die. So long have we been away from our Limitless Way of Being—Life Everlasting—that even the Earth's most holy tribal teachings have us believing that the Circle of Life includes the death of humanity before they can experience Heaven. It is one of the biggest lies we ever bought.

When you recognize that God has a plan for you to become more conscious and masterful again, to regain your Divinity again, it is really very easy to become your own doctor, to **become your own healing authority**. Once you get this, you want to learn several strategies so you can become masterful enough to know and trust that **YOU CAN HEAL ANYTHING** that you create in your school of learning—your body-mind. When this is in place, you have your own hospital and your own pharmacy . (Your body is the greatest pharmacy in the world and your body-mind beats the Library of Congress any day. It knows everything!).

Being your own doctor or healing authority does not mean that you have to do this alone. You can call on alternative healthcare professionals who are masterful in what they know and do. As a matter of fact when you are in senility, you cannot do it alone. So don't even try. There is nothing to prove here. Get rid of stubborn, stupid pride. You are only delaying your pleasure and your healing.

Above and beyond this, **you have to trust yourself and God-Goddess**—since all healing comes from Them. Even if you drop the ball and lose faith, They never go away, even when we abandon ourselves or shut Them out or off. We are impatient...They are not. They don't even expect us to get it this lifetime. Thank goodness They Are Infinite Patience with us little whippersnappers.

When I made the decision to become my own doctor after the experience with the rheumatologist, I did not have clearly formulated the understandings that I now have. What I did have was the Divine Intelligence within me, tenderly and lovingly whispering to me to "get" that there was another way. Actually there are a lot of other ways.

Thru the years, I have come to really trust that inner knowing. My faith really tested itself with the senility. I fell back on myself many times and I never quit. I remember meeting with Leonard and Isabelle Orr in Santa Fe right before a week long training that they were going to do in September of 1999.

I was thrilled to get to see them…it was not planned. The first thing Leonard said to me was that I looked better than the letter I had sent him a few weeks previously—I had been pretty down.

At that meeting, a few other folks asked Leonard what he had done to get thru senility. Leonard replied "Hundreds of things". I could relate; Kel and I did bunches of different herbs, tinctures, diets, supplements, soil based organisms, white powder gold, colloidal silver, all of Dr. Schulze's products continuously including the Incurables Program, the Rife machine, juice fasts, fasting, Massage, Reiki, tons of B.E.S.T., tons of processing, etc., etc., etc., plus a daily regimen of other strategies which were many and varied.

It may seem inconsistent that at the emotional-mental level, I work with myself and others identifying "the problem" to address and then not go to a doctor to get a diagnosis to find out what specific dis-eases I was going thru in senility. It may seem so to another. To me what I was doing was totally consistent.

You see, the dis-ease—whatever label you put on it—is not the problem. Cancer, Aids, arthritis, poverty, etc. are not the culprit; they are merely the symptom. Just as a subluxation of the vertebrae is merely a symptom of what is going on in the body-mind. These are manifestations (the effects, if you will) of thought forms—habits of belief, conditioned habits of feelings and emotions.

When you identify the thought-decision-belief-feeling-emotion, then you can address the cause of your condition-experience. You will want to address it with a technology that can convert the causal material into energy and light. Talking about it will not change it. Getting an "aha" will not change it. Medication, chemotherapy, radiation, drugs and surgery will not change it.

You must work with the information at a level that is beyond rational, logical thought. **Rational thought has nothing to do with healing**. Rebirthing, Quantum Dynamics, Body Electronics, B.E.S.T. Chiropractic (especially Level Three Dialogue) work with you at this level. Faith is a strategic instrument for us, as is prayer. Be willing to see that God has given us these other instruments of healing as a higher form of prayer.

What these technologies do is help you not only "reframe" the thought forms, emotions and feelings, they also change the chemistry in your body. New neural pathways are created and your physiology alters, creating new understanding and new ways of being. These technologies take the emotional charge out that formerly held you hostage in your own body-mind. They also release the denial, hiding and withholding of energy; the patterns of conditioning get released, converting you into a different person—a person of renewed vision.

There are a number of healing modalities that support us in feeling better in our bodies when we get conscious of painful memories. Some of these methods, while they seem to create resolution, actually do nothing more than create suppression of our feelings which creates superficial healing at best. The Sedona Method and Neuro-Linguistic Programming are such modalities.

The Chinese do not work with diagnosis as Western Doctors do. They work with what is going on in the body; they work to rebalance and harmonize the body according to their findings. This strategy feels like an intelligent way to work with the sacredness of the body. There is an honoring that goes on in the Orient that the Western world has not awakened to as yet.

While Kel and I do not know the specific names of all the dis-eases I went thru, (I had over 50 different symptoms—many at any given time), we do know I went thru four terminal dis-eases that my body could identify. As my body-mind revealed the thought forms-beliefs-decisions-emotions and feelings, we addressed them one by one.

13) OOPS! I MISSED THE MARK

Did you know that in Aramaic (the language that Jesus spoke when he was here two thousand years ago), the definition for "sin" was "Oops, I missed the mark"? Well, I apparently did this very thing with regard to my hip...

I went to have my hip x-rayed three months after I fell. I was horrified to see that the trochanter head while attached to the neck of the femur was off by 22 and 1/2 millimeters. When I fell, the first x-ray showed only a 5 millimeter difference. While Innate had attached the bone, it had not done a very good job, in my opinion. I was really disappointed and angry, especially since I had continually asked my MAP Team and Source if the bones were in their right place. They continually said, "Yes, it is in its right place".

At one point, my MAP Team questioned my continuously questioning them with regard to the bones and their right placement. "Wasn't I trusting them?" My fears, I thought had been appeased. So when I took my MAP Team to task about the x-ray and consequences of all this, they told me I had opportunity to address my fears and my own lack of trust.

So I began a process of "rectifying my error"...of repenting for my lack of trust. I threw myself into the old conditioning...thinking I must have done wrong...been insufficient in my faith...been unworthy to receive my good...I got caught up in victim thought again. "God-Goddesss, will I ever be done with this"? " Yes"!!! "When"? "When you get bored with it"!

Needless to say, my confidence in the MAP Team was greatly diminished. I am not certain I have healed this yet with them. And I realize that this is a reflection of my own lack of faith in self and my relationship to Source.

Kel and I know how to move bones. We have done it before with other people. We know the bone will move, although it has not moved to date—even though each time we have asked, we have gotten confirmation that it has shifted some.

Kel assures me that my body has a lot of other priorities right now. Again, I feel like I am testing my faith. I know with most of my being that we can create right time-right place for this trochanter head. I just have to get my trust-faith to 100%.

The same holds true for my hands, which have become misshapen, stiff, degenerated and very arthritic in the last three years. With 100% belief-trust-faith in the amazing healing grace of this body-mind, Source and I can heal my hands and even my left foot to be useful and strong again.

One of my friends used to say my hands were like steel, they were so strong when I would give her shoulder, back and neck tune-ups. Being a Registered Massage Therapist was an occupation of love. I want to have that as a part of my life experience again.

And I want to be able to dance again and walk and run without a limp and without pain and stress in my body from having to compensate for a body out of kilter. I choose to have even legs and I choose to have this occur easily, gently and gracefully. I can create this. I know how. Our bodies and our minds can do as we request, as we affirm these things for ourselves in consciousness. As I decide this and put my attention on this, I create this and only this and I am grateful.

I am grateful Mother-Father God for this Living Temple, for this Life and for the Sacred Breath that resides within me. Support me into regeneration and youthing; that I may grow into my Seed of Greatness and Limitless Physical Perfection and Freedom and Heaven On Earth in this Body Now!

14) UNDERSTANDINGS AND TOOLS FOR HEALING

When we "max out", "go the limit" in senility and death, and we have had the mind set that we can outwit them (outlast them), we reach a point where we can come back without resistance. We are not coming back to our old "selves", because we will never be the same again. We have burned away the conditioning that formulated our former "selves"…the dross as Anna Lee would say. We have a cleaner, more creative presence that has more unity and more clarity. It is almost like we have had the near death experience and we come back into ourselves with a tremendous passion for life and an insistence to share it with others.

What follows are many understandings I had before I went into this, awesome revelations given during the process and the magnificent, strategic tools that Source gifted me, to do not only senility and death with, but life as well.

15) DEFENSE PHYSIOLOGY
PART I

Structurally we haven't changed much since what we call "cave man" days. Our physiology (which is how our body functions) has remained essentially the same as well. Back then, when one of our relatives came to find himself nose to nose with a sabertooth tiger, rest assured that the bodily functions of our kin were maxed out by the fright.

Maxed out means that his breathing stopped and then diminished if he chose to fight, and accelerated if he chose to run. The very same thing occurred with his heart rate and blood pressure. His abdomen, anus, neck, all of his musculature and bodily functions momentarily tightened and rigidified. For all practical purposes his physiology shut down for that moment creating an imprint (memory) which we all carry today.

All of the above and similar experiences happened many times, creating the imprints of conditioned fear, terror and paranoia within us. This has been carried through the millenia in our DNA, accumulating more and more of like conditioned reaction/ responses. So much so, that even the perceived notion of possible danger triggers this same primal response.

This imprint in our physiology has come to be accepted as normal function. We are definitely not relaxed and as such, we are not aware of how tightly strung we are. In essence we are constantly on guard, defended and don't even recognize it. It is almost as though the inherited mindset expects that sabertooth tiger at any moment.

With this much perpetual unconscious overload, we are set up for creating dysfunction and dis-ease. We think that how we are, is the way we were meant to be…and that is not even the truth of our being. This situation is real, it exists. It is not right, it is not wrong. It is our history and it creates our biology.

The way that we have accelerated ourselves technologically but not emotionally, has created a lifestyle that is fast paced and burdened with a myriad of stressful activities. As a result, we live anticipating saber-tooth tigers at every turn. We are poised in adrenal overload, poised in defense physiology and we don't even know it.

This is readily understood by the recognition that it takes an incredible amount of effort and discipline to quiet the mind's chatter and to really relax the body. Most people don't even consider that they can do this. We live in unconscious overload, constricted aliveness and duressed bodily function.

There are many tools to change this and to increase your conscious awareness around this. They will be mentioned at the end of part two on defense physiology.

16) DEFENSE PHYSIOLOGY
PART II

The previous article on Defense Physiology dealt with primordial mankind. This article deals with the subject as it relates to contemporary society.

First of all, what is defense physiology? Well, obviously it is a state of the body being defended and in this case, a state that the person is not even aware of. This is because we, generally speaking, are born in or into this condition. Many of us experienced defense physiology before we were even born through our mother. At any time during our intra-uterine development, if our mother believed she was going to be injured physically or emotionally, whether it happened or not, we received the chemical message as well as the emotional message and the imprint was made.

This was not the original imprint. It was simply a replay of memory of our primal ancestors and before. Each time these imprints occur, our experience locks us into believing in the "no exit terror" of past pain and trauma. These imprints of injury, real or perceived, become a pattern that affect us the rest of this lifetime. Enough imprinting and we experience difficulties in relationships, jobs, finance, and eventually bodily function.

Defense physiology usually manifests early in life as a form of insecurity, the need for someone or something to cover up our denied belief in the separation from Mother Father God, called something else. These are often labeled as dis-eases like alcohol or other addictions, and a myriad of other names. The psychology and psychiatry books are full of labels. (They teach labeling as a "fine" art.)

This imprinted information is not carved in stone, nor is it wrong. It is only memory.

And memory is something you volunteered for, so that you could learn from it, heal it and teach others about it. Without this understanding, we are left with blaming one or both our parents, ourselves, others and nothing heals.

Our opportunity is to indeed learn from where we are, make the desired life supportive changes and get on with enjoying more of our lives. There are many tools and they all work. There are wonderful workshops where one can work on issues with others or in counseling one on one.

Initially, the defense physiology from a healer's perspective is seen as an attitude or in the body or both. Often the body is fairly easy to teach to relax. However teaching the mind is a little more difficult. This is because the mind sees the defendedness as a form of protection and there is a fear that if it is given up, death will quickly follow. Of course this isn't true.

Consequently, many therapists only work the surface or near surface issues for fear of the powerful death urge the individual may bring up. (Isn't liability an amazing concept?). The truth is most professionals do not even know about this and have not gone here themselves; they are therefore, unable to support their client in their core issues. As a consequence, the therapist can only take the client as far as they themselves have been willing to go.

When the client is approached with tools of empowerment and shown how they are safe, by a facilitator who has gone deep into their own process, wonderful things can and do happen for the individual and the Collective since WE ARE ALL ONE.

The client has to be encouraged and shown how they can master their imprinting regardless of their fear of what they may find. Birth trauma may seem insignificant and birth trauma is where it begins until they are willing and ready to go back to Origin. These are the imprints we have come into this lifetime to heal. They are the foundation for everything else that has happened or continues to happen to us.

Listed below are a variety of tools that support one out of defense physiology and into conscious awareness of their energy and their potential. These strategies are by no means the only tools that accomplish this. They are the ways we have found here at A Next Step…light center for emotional healing to be the most successful and we use them all the time. These are not necessarily in any order of preference or potency. They all work.

1. Twenty Connected Breaths and the Basic Thought Meditation
2. Rebirthing or Conscious Energy Breath
3. BEST Chiropractic
4. Body Electronics
5. The Light Bridge Attunement
6. The Sweeping Breath
7. Quantum Dynamics
   a. Eagle's Breath
   b. Q.D.Statement
   c. Magnetic Statement
8. Spiritual Purification
9. Bursting the Body Light—Violet Flame of Forgiveness Breath/Meditation
10. Three in One—Body Mind, Spirit
11. Aromatherapy Hands On Healing
12. Environmental Accupuncture
13. Vision Quest
14. Massage
15. Reiki (and more)

To learn about these strategies check out our web site at **http://www.anextstep.org** or email us at: kelley@anextstep.org

17) PAIN

Pain is a sorely misunderstood emotion. It is the most valuable messenger that we have; it is one way that our body communicates with us. It is how our body gets our attention. It says to us "Hey! Look here. Please see what's going on here." Yet, **We fear pain and we fear our bodies in pain**. And we fear feeling just about anything at all in our bodies.

When we reach for aspirin and pain killers to quash the pain without figuring out what's going on, we kill the messenger. We make the pain wrong and our bodies wrong. We become frightened that something is wrong…when really something is just communicating what is. Our body is talking to us, getting our attention the best way it knows how.

We have not been trained to listen or even been able to interpret the bodies' language. We are so frightened of ourselves and frightened of feeling ourselves. If we would just chill out and talk to our bodies, we would learn an enormous amount about ourselves and the goings on of our physiology.

So, how about this? How about be willing to start communicating with your heart, colon, kidneys, liver, eyes, blood, etc. You might be surprised and pleased with your interactions. All you have to do is decide to. If you get nothing, try again and again. Know that this communication is possible. The only thing stopping it is your own "unbelief". So suspend that and go for it. You have nothing to lose and everything to gain.

I remember Rebirthing a young woman (age 25) some years ago. I asked her to ask her body about something. I was surprised when she screamed. She got frightened because she didn't know her body could talk to her…it did.

What I have come to realize about pain is that pain is nothing more than extreme tension in the body. We are all tense. **We are all defended against life**. As that tension continues and increases, it's hold (in varying parts of the body, depending on what we are defending against) becomes pain.

So the key to addressing all pain—from the heavy duty kind (Cancer, Aids, etc.) to muscular discomfort (from overwork or a good workout at the gym) is relaxation.

Most people can't relax; they don't know how. Visualization, Meditation, Yoga, Tai Chi, Chi Gung, Massage, Reiki are excellent avenues for teaching the body how to let go, harmonize and be pain free. Each of these must be done as a practice (done regularly, as in daily) in order to have any long lasting effect.

Rebirthing, Quantum Dynamics, B.E.S.T. Chiropractic, Body Electronics will not only relax you, they will also release the thought forms—decisions, judgements, habits of belief-feelings-emotions-experiences and conditions which created the reaction of defense and thus the tension and pain.

When you learn to embrace the pain, it really talks to you. When I fell, lots of issues came to consciousness for address. I processed all day, everyday nonstop for several weeks. When the pain presented itself, I got to address what created the pain in thought—feeling with Q.D., then I used lobelia (an excellent anti-spasmodic; spasm-tension reliever). I felt happy to be moving so much material into energy and light.

When we stop running away from the pain within ourselves; when we face the messenger and the particular part of the body from which the pain originates, we can address the programs—thought forms-feelings we agreed to heal this lifetime in this body. This will teach us something of why we are here; it will lend awareness to our reason or purpose for being. Pain truly is our ally and when we fully recognize this, we will know to take advantage of the fact that **PAIN IS THE DOORWAY TO CONSCIOUSNESS.**

It is nearly inconceivable how much pain our body-mind is capable of generating and then holding. Sometimes that pain feels far larger than the body it is being held in. There have been times when the pain within me felt like it not only filled up my being, but also the room and building that I was in.

I remember one such day. Kelley had just finished working on me and had left to run some errands. I was lying on the massage table in our workroom. I was feeling sorry for myself because of the pain and my circumstance. I was feeling victim and caged up.

Suddenly, I heard a most strange sound running the length of our house. The sound then came into the room I was in. It came in along the floor, under the massage table. It felt most odd. I sat up and got up to see what it could possibly be. I looked everywhere around on the floor. When I moved my vision to the window sill, I saw the most precious tiny brown bird—she could not have been more than 2 inches tall.

I'm certain she was just as surprised to see me, as I was to hear her flutterings within my home. As I began talking to her to tell her that she was safe, she flew out of the room. I went to the front door to open it so she could fly out. I looked for her all over, as I talked to her to soothe her. Then, I heard the back door blow open. She must have flown out as unexpectedly as she flew in.

God is so great. It was as if She was saying to me: "Release Yourself! Uncage yourself! You are the one who got you into this. You are the one who will get yourself out of it. Undo it...it's easy." I felt better by far. I smile every time I think of this experience and of how much God loves me.

18) CONTROL

Most of us live with a White Knuckle Death Grip on Life. We are defended, contracted, tense, holding on like crazy, which is one reason Americans spend over $500 million on laxatives annually. (Sunrider International, 1997). We fool ourselves thinking we are in control of our lives. The truth is we are not in control of much, but the Universe is compassionate with us.

We are really pretty funny. We ask for change, then when it starts materializing, we put on the skids. I did this so many times. I tried "stopping the snowball, because I thought it was going down the hill too fast". Mom and Dad God would always laugh at me. When They got me to realize it was only my thought that it was going too fast, I could relax, let go and "it" slowed down remarkably.

Letting go of control has everything to do with healing all dis-ease and dysfunction, including senility and the infancy consciousness locked in trauma in our bodies. Lots of people are so tense and defended that they don't know how to let go, relax and surrender.

We control as much of our being as we possibly can. Anything that is within our ability to contract, hold back on, we do it. We have learned that our body's natural functions are absolutely wrong. As a consequence, we hold back coughing, sneezing, burping, farting. We even hold back our urine and fecal flow…til it is convenient. Holding back our natural functions, stops our energy, toxifies our system and creates devastating effects. It is almost like we fear what our bodies do and are. How can this be natural?

I remember reading about Marcel Mastrianni ,the handsome leading man in the film "Fanny". He told the interviewer that he would never get married because he could not imagine the shame he would have to go through with his beloved if he were to happen to "expell gas in her presence". Good God! I noticed that he was appearing quite aged. Yes! holding back your gas...a natural function of your beautiful body can age you!

We also learn very young that it is wrong to express how we feel. We learn that crying and being sad are wrong. We learn that being afraid is wrong. And there is or has been no one in our lives to tell us otherwise, because everyone around us is as closed down—if not more so. There are a huge number of folks who are greatly fearful and angry who would absolutely deny this, because their prozac has them believing life is wonderful.

We especially learn that anger and rage are wrong, because it frightens us. So we make sure, we squash those feelings. And if anger and rage happen to spill out into our consciousness, we make real sure we deny that that is how we feel. We are expert at avoidance and masterful actors...and boy do we know how to pretend.

AND...we can pretend all we want. Many of us are so sentient, that we develop habits to bury the sentiency, because no one has taught us about it and it feels like more than we can handle. This is why there are so many addictive habits and so many addicts on the planet. We hide our feelings and we hide from our feeling nature.

We are energy and energy loves to move. We were made to cry and laugh, to fart, burp and poop. We were made to feel and express. Instead of being thoughtful, expressive, flowing creations of God, we have become domesticated, held back robots. We are numb, shut down, unconscious and as far away from our nature and our beginnings as we have ever been.

Most of our decisions and actions around life come from our white knuckle death grip; our old conditioned fear, terror and paranoia around life. As such, we seek to control our lives by continuously stopping our energy; we think this will keep us safe. In the long run, there is a price to pay for this conscious habit gone unconscious. After a while, it becomes killing anxiety, inexplicable nervousness, depression, unhappiness, lethargy, short life and early death.

So what we must do is learn new systems of control that do not stop our energy; that involve letting go of the white knuckle death grip. Quantum Dynamics and Rebirthing are great for this. By utilizing the energy that is Q.D. and the sacred breath within us, we learn to surrender in the middle of everything. By doing this, we gain energy, more light and conscious awareness of our feeling nature and our situation. We get to direct our energy and our lives without fear; we get to be at choice.

19) DANCING WITH DEATH

The notion of death for many of us is a chilling experience. Chilling and frightening because we fear it so. No doubt because our bodies remember the circumstances of the many times we have died. And because many of us did not remember that we are love, the way we left was pretty awful and unloving. Having this much terror and fear associated with the memories, makes just about everything far worse (in our minds).

Each time we give up the will to live, we experience fragmentation—probably from the fright of the experience. Our body-mind probably freaks out and shatters like a mirror. This creates more work for us as we seek to become whole again, for we must then retrieve those parts of self back to ourselves. God calls this "lost will" that fragments away. (Ceanne DeRohan, Original Cause).

In the years of senility that I have experienced, Death and I tangoed a lot. The first year and a half were the deadliest. I had lost most of my personal power and strength, and my fears were all consuming. As a result, Death led the dance. I felt at NO CHOICE and consequently powerless.

Despite the feeling of powerlessness, I fought tooth and nail to maintain—to stay alive. Death is a formidable opponent when we give our power to it. The challenge is not to. As with any energy in the Universe, whatever we put our attention on, we call to ourselves.

However, if we know nothing of Death or we seek to avoid it (as a result of our denied fears), it will eclipse us. If we make it wrong (by running away from it) or we make it right (using it as an insurance policy when our lives become too challenging or conflicted), we are giving it power over us.

We must seek to know Death, be willing to look it in the eye, converse with it, so we can make intelligent choices with regard to it and our relationship to it. We can do this without marrying it. We can do this without dying.

As a persona, Death is usually portrayed ghoulishly as in the Grim Reaper. Sometimes, however, in some mythologies, Death takes on a regal portrayal as in the <u>Vedas</u>. The Vedas are some of the oldest scriptures of India. (Perhaps millions of years old). Each of the four Vedas are divided into two parts: 1) work and 2) knowledge. It is this second part called the <u>Upanishads</u> from which I wish to tell you the story of Death. Upanishad translates to "secret teaching which destroys the bonds of ignorance and leads to the ultimate goal of freedom".

In this particular Upanishad it is revealed that "The secret of immortality is to be found in purification of the heart, in meditation, in realization of the identity of the Self within and Brahman without, for Immortality is Union with God". (<u>The Wisdom of the Hindu Mystics, The Upanishads, Breath of Life</u>, Swami Prabhavananda and Frederick Manchester).

The story is about a man named Vajasraba. He is hoping for divine favor, so he has been asked to perform a rite which requires that he give away all of his possessions. Instead of offering his finest possessions, he offers his most useless possessions. His young son Natchiketa observing this, thinks his father's action is "doomed to utter darkness". So the boy says to his father, "To whom givest thou me?" At first, his father gives no response, but with persistence, his father at last says "I give you to Death".

The child, seemingly of more integrity than his father, journeys to the house of the Lord of Death—Yama. He finds Death not at home and he waits. He waits three nights. When at last the Lord of Death returns, he grants Natchiketa three boons, one for each night that he waited.

The first wish that his father receive him in love when he returns is easily granted. The second that Yama teach him the fire ceremony that leads people to heaven, is not only granted, but Yama decides to name the ceremony after the boy: Natchiketa Sacrifice. The third boon is not given so readily. It takes a great deal of persistance on the boy's part to get Yama to consent, because even the gods could not learn it from him. At last Yama agrees to teach him the secrets of Immortality.

The information that the Lord of Death shares with Natchiketa feels like teachings that have been given by mystics, gurus, rishis of long ago and from the New Age. This tells me that this information and wisdom have been with us all along. We simply have not been able to hear it or take action on it...probably because we have not been ready.

Yama says "To the thoughtless...deceived by the vanity of earthly possessions who believe that this world alone is real, will they fall again and again birth after birth into my jaws and to them, the path that leads to the eternal abode is not revealed". He says blessed are they who seek the Eternal Life.

Yama says, "He who has discrimination, whose mind is steady and whose heart is pure, reaches the goal and having reached it is born no more". He talks about the supports and ways that one may achieve Union with the Divine. He talks about the use and knowledge of the mantra Om, meditation, use of Spiritual Purification and aligning with the inner self to gain Union with Brahman.

The boy Natchiketa was freed from all impurities, from death and was united with Brahman. Natchiketa surrendered himself to the truth of the Self...that the Self and Brahman (God) are One. "Thus will it be for another also if he know the innermost self".

Death as presented thru the great teacher Don Juan Matus (as revealed through his apprentice Carlos Castaneda in the book <u>Journey to Ixtlan: the Lessons of Don Juan</u>), is a valuable advisor on our earthly sojourn. Don Juan says that Death is our eternal companion. It is always to our left at an arm's length. He says that it is always watching us and always will, until the day that it taps us (takes us).

Don Juan says we can call on our death at any time for advice and that Death will whisper into our ear. Its advice and warnings come as a chill to our body. Don Juan feels that we can get rid of a lot of our self importance and pettiness when our Death is our advisor. When we accept this, we cut thru the world of Maya much quicker. Death helps us "cut thru the crap" as Don Juan would say.

"Without an awareness of death, everything is ordinary, trivial. It is only because death is stalking us that the world is an unfathomable mystery"...."Having to believe that the world is mysterious and unfathomable was the expression of a warrior's innermost predilection. Without it, he had nothing". (Tales of Power, Carlos Castaneda)

"In a world where death is the hunter, there is not time for regrets or doubts. There is only time for decisions". Death can absolutely humble us and make us wise beyond our years. When we fear Death, we make it wrong and run from it. We whine, whimper and act as sheep. In this running, there is no respect for the Self; there is nothing but spent energy.

Death can teach us a lot when we are in body and we are awake to it. If we are asleep, we become victimized by our own ignorance; by our own mind. When we are impeccable in our decisions and in how we live, Death honors that impeccability and supports us to learn more.

In order to be impeccable, we must know about the death urge. Death urge has a life of its own within us. It is almost like it has been hard wired into our psyches. The death urge according to Leonard Orr is "a psychic entity that has an intelligence and a life urge, and as such it resists change. It's goal is to destroy the body or separate the Life and soul from the body." It will kill us because this is its purpose...unless we kill it first.

The way that we kill the death urge within us is by changing our thoughts and feelings alchemically within our body-mind. We do this one emotional thought at a time...until it has no more power over us.

It is essential that we become conscious of our death urge and heal it before someone in our families acts it out.

Pets and children are often the first ones in families to act out the death urge of family traditions. They will do emotional, physical, mental symptoms in the form of accidents or dis-ease, and if no one gets it, they will do death. It is their way of extending the life of their parent or grandparent. They do not know that this will not save their relative and it is done unconsciously.

"Some people can't even begin to heal their family death urge until their parents die, because it is not in our awareness. It is not active in our mind or emotions. When it does become active, it causes people to indulge in self-sabotaging behavior…we sabotage personal, business or career decisions, develop bad or unproductive habits, have accidents, etc. We feel depressed and hopeless. Obviously suicidal or homocidal dreams or feelings and thoughts are a sign of the unconscious death urge taking over our lives."

"The death urge is easy to detect: loss of appetite or eating too much because it is the only thing meaningful or pleasurable to do, depression and discouragement, suicidal thoughts, violent dreams, no interests nor goals, etc.". (Conscious Connection, The newsletter of Rebirth International "The Death Urge",Leonard Orr, Sept., 2001).

We can absolutely heal the death urge within us. The first thing is to get conscious of it. **If you are in the death process or senility, you must decide continuously to outlive it**. Ways to do this have been spoken of throughout this book and will be ennumerated in Chapters 23-34.

When you heal the death urge that you have learned from your family, you can relearn it from friends, lovers, co-workers, clients, other relatives, etc. When this happens, you can use the same methods of healing to undo it again. Continue unraveling it, until you have total body-mind mastery over it.

For those who are unconvinced that Union with God is where we are headed; for those who still believe in Separation—that Heaven is some place outside of us, please hear this: **You cannot achieve God consciousness without a body**. As we continually succomb to old habits of killing our bodies, we distance ourselves from achieving Union with God.

We all create how we are going to die—whether we are conscious of it or not. Our moment by moment decisions every day create movement and matter towards these deaths. As such, **all death is suicide**.

Knowing this and being awake to this habit from the past, we can choose and take action to do otherwise. Knowing that death has been and is what other people may choose, **we can choose instead Union with God in these bodies now**. It is a decision which will have to be remade often and action on it will have to be taken daily.

20) LIGHT AT THE END OF THE TUNNEL

The following are some poems that came as I saw and embraced the Light at the end of the tunnel.

AWAKEN!
Never give up! Do you hear me!
Never give up! Do I say!
I pledge in this precious moment to the Divinity of the Sacred Trust within me now:
In Your Image and Likeness I Am That I Am! I Am That I Am! I Am That I Am!
Bhole Baba Ki Jai!
Jai Maha Maya Ki Jai!
Jagadambe Mata Ki Jai!

MOTHER STRENGTH
We are the Earth; her precious land.
We are the Earth; her vital waters.
We are her creatures large and small.
We are her majesty and beauty,
......her courage and strength.
Mother Earth reclaims her Power and Divinity
......as she purifies her bodies.
She knows what she does, for she has done it before

.......masterfully.
Grateful am I to have the fortitude to do the same.

BE IT
Pure Thought.
Pure Breath.
Pure Being.
Pure Joy.
Pure Ease.
Pure Song.
We are the chalice of Spirit and Will, Body and Heart.
Come along. Come along. Come along.

I AM THAT WHICH I DECIDE TO BECOME
I am Divine; I am the Goddess.
 (do I matter?)
I am Divine; I am the Goddess.
 (do You care?)
I am Divine; I am the Goddess.
 (can You hear me?)
I am Divine; I am the Goddess.
 (can You see me?)
You are Divine; You are the Goddess.
 (how come I feel like a brown spot?)
You are Divine; You are the Goddess.
 (how come I hurt so much?)
You are Divine; You are the Goddess.
 (how can I let go?)
DECIDE! You are Divine; You are the Goddess.
OK............I am Divine; I am the Goddess.

Yes.........I Am Divine; I Am the Goddess.
YES!...I definitely Am Divine; I Am the Goddess.

LEARNING TO RECEIVE
I take from you these gifts you offer.
  They are a blessing.
I take from you your shoulder to cry on.
  I am grateful.
I take from you your willingness to be here.
  I am humbled.
I take from you your words of encouragement.
  It is a reminder.
I take from you your love and constancy.
  I am worthy. Jai Ma!

I AM
Solar Christ Presence,
   Blaze thru me the Phoenix Rising..
      to its Limitless Star of Perfection.
Behold. I Am Ascended and Translated into the Eternal Peace
      of Earth, Air , Water , Fire and The Ethers.
And so it is.

GLORY TO THE MOTHER
Kwan Yin, bless you for your compassion in loving this body.
Green Tara, bless you for your patience in keeping me strong of faith.
Kali, bless you for your endurance in destroying the sewer of my mind.
Chamunda, bless you for your ruthlessness and unwillingness to yield.
   Glory to the Mother in all of Her forms within me.

Blessed be the fullness of Her Breath within my lungs.

Blessed be Her pure sweet nectar coursing my veins.

May Manna be my substance and Love be my eternal function.

Blessed Be to The Mother in all Her Forms…for all that I Am Is Goddess.

SEED OF GREATNESS

Yikes! Do you see her soaring?

Goodness…have you ever seen her so grand?

The Goddess is alive within me now!

Victory to the Deva in all her magnificence!

[1]"She keeps me upright and dispels all darkening darkness.

She gives me knowledge with a Mother's wisest sense.

She dispels all my fears, pain and illusion.

She helps me traverse the Oceans of Life."

She is my Core; She is my guiding Light.

She lifts me higher and higher into

Realms of Ease and Perfection.

In Her, I soar and thru Her I am made grand.

Thank you Mahendra Baba

---

1.   from Mother Aarati

21) GOD IS NOT A PICTURE

Somewhere along the way we have gotten the idea that God is some energy that we can put in a box or in a statue or in a picture. I think we got to be this way as we learned to defend ourselves in all relationships. To provide "safety" for ourselves, we depersonalized everything and everybody. God does not stop or stand still any more than any other energy in the Universe.

The marvelous thing about the Universe is that it is constantly changing, which means that everything is constantly experiencing flux and movement. The Main Mover cannot hold still while It directs the evolution of the Entire Cosmos.

I find it most exciting and stabilizing to know God is evolving as I evolve or rather that I get to evolve as God-Goddess evolve. I look forward to experiencing the fullness of God in the diversity of humanity as we ascend into Union; as it is accepted by humanity that man is Divine, that we are God. For then Harmony, Understanding and Cooperation will abound.

As a child I was raised to believe that God is a picture which to my young mind meant that God did not change; He was always the same kind of God. I learned from the St. Joseph nuns at St. Augustine elementary that God is a formidable (fire and brimstone) force to be reckoned with. I feared God the Father as a child; Jesus was my solace and Mother Mary was my comforter.

I was also raised to believe that my God—the Catholic God was better and different from the God of Lutherans, Methodists, Buddists, Muslims etc. I was also taught that all the poor black babies in Africa that were orphans and without a Catholic Church to attend or Catholic God to save them were in a lot of trouble.

My relationship to God as a child was one dimensional, probably because I was one dimensional. They all (God , Jesus and Mary) felt flat to me…until the night that Mary appeared to me. And I soon forgot that event altogether until years later.

As a result of getting my way—to not have to attend parochial school any longer—I was in the third grade—(I do not know how on earth I pulled that one off—Spirit must have really been looking out for me! All my brothers and sister had to continue going to parochial school), I had to attend catechism. I did this obediently until junior high school.

When the priests and nuns refused to answer my questions about evolution versus creation theory, I started playing hooky from catechism class. How could it be that there are things that we are not supposed to know? At the time I thought the nuns were holding back on me. Now I realize that they probably had no clue.

As a consequence of this event, I decided to become an atheist. I felt what this was like for a while and then became an agnostic. I maintained this for a number of years. My parents—especially my Mom was angry at me when I refused to marry in the Catholic Church. I was not willing however, to compromise; I had to be true to myself. I now recognize my stubborness.

I married an atheist who had been raised Wisconsin Synod Lutheran. For our wedding, we compromised and had a Congregational minister marry us. We raised our son sans any religious orientation and I wonder how this has affected his valuing of life. I know he has a good work ethic and is a great person, I just don't know if he believes in God.

As I matured, I softened my disposition toward God. I learned a lot about myself, God and my relationshp with Them as I began my path to healing which started when my marriage started falling apart in

1975. Isn't that the way? When we come apart, we seek a Higher Understanding. Or maybe we seek to be understood.

I found out thru Rebirthing that I had quite a lot of anger with Father God and I had a lot of unforgiveness with Jesus. I also found out I misplaced this anger on a lot of my relationships. I remember my son saying to me when he was about seven, "Gosh Mom, you are always angry". Breathwork and Q.D. have helped me in healing this.

I met Babaji of Hairakhan in 1981 or '82 thru Paramahansa Yogananda in Autobiography of a Yogi. I met Him in spirit in 1985 at my first Aarati (sanscrit for Celebration for Lights written for Babaji and us, by Mahendra Baba). This Aarati happened the same weekend as my Quantum Dynamics initiation.

I started crying as the Aarati began and I did not know why. I closed my eyes as the music continued, to find Babaji standing right in front of me with His arms outstretched waiting to enfold me. He said, "Welcome home daughter." My soul remembered the Aarati and Baba, even though I did not. I sobbed like a baby throughout the ceremony. Babaji has been in my heart since then. He is my inspiration and a constant in my life.

I knew about Mother God when I was young. I figured it out. How could God not be male and female, if we were made in Their image and likeness? I did not have a personal relationship with Mother God though, until I started processing the Ceanne DeRohan Will books. Or rather until I allowed the information in the books to process me in 1985 on into and thru the 1990's.

As I read thru the books, they took me thru quite a lela. They really explain a lot of what is happening on Earth and what it is we have opportunity to heal within ourselves and in all our relationships. I freaked out one day with the question: '"What if I don't like who Mother God is?" As I cleaned up the reflections, I realized She is me and I love me.

I love the Goddess in all of Her attributes and qualities. I love her Will Body, Her Creative Expression, Her Tolerance. I love Her willingness to manifest and birth us. I love Her compassion, ruthlessness and incredible patience with us. The Goddess has an understanding and experience of Creation that has taken the other parts of God a long time to get. I trust Humanity will get it soon.

God-Goddess have many faces and attributes just as diverse as the reflections on planet Earth now. They do not care which aspects of Themselves we resonate with. They do, however, wish us to open to receive Them, because we are a part of Them and belief in Separation must end. Denial of our true essence, our true nature will not be tolerated any longer.

WE ALL ARE ONE. WE ARE ALL GOD-GODDESS. And for this planet to be free of all unnaturalness, all belief and participation in Separation, all belief and participation in being disconnected from God, we must accept and acknowledge that WE ALL ARE ONE. We must acknowledge and accept this in all that we are, in order to ascend into the Higher Thought-Understanding-Feeling- Being of our God-hood.

When we accept and embrace this with every electron of our being, dis-ease, aging, poverty, lack, war, victim consciousness will be the only things of our experience that have gone extinct. When we accept and embrace our Goddesshood, we will be better human beings than we have been in a long time. We will also once again Have all and Be all that God-Goddess Are and Have. We will Be One With All That Is. We Will Be Magnificent and Divine. Such deliciousness I seek to embrace within me now.

As more of us get this truth and take action with it daily in our lives, our Union will create unstoppable good, harmony, understanding, peace and abundance throughout the Cosmos. Remember energy loves to move....we are not a still frame.

You can choose to have a very personal relationship with God. The way you have one is to decide. Start talking to God—the God-Goddess within. It does not need to be a formalized prayer. Just start talking. It is being heard. As you are willing to empty yourself of your old programming, you will create places within to hear Them. I call Them, Mom and Dad because I choose to be this personal with Them.

22) A BIT HASTY?

When I recognized that I could release information—matter—density from my being, I was like a maniac. I wanted to "get rid of it all right now!" I did not understand about energy and I did not understand that the Universe gives us exactly what we ask for. I especially knew nothing about compassion for the self. I was for all purposes, reckless in my petitions to the Universe to release "my stuff" all at once.

I made this request on four different occasions. (I am a slow learner). The first time was the first day of training to be a Q.D. Teacher in June of 1990. The training made me face some pretty ugly unconscious conditioning and long hidden fears. It felt like what I think Marine boot camp must be like. I was really hard on myself, so my reflections were rather harsh. I cried a lot and felt dread each morning when I awoke to find I was still there. I wanted so to have it be a bad dream. And I wanted it to be over. In retrospect, it was the best thing that could have happened—I was a wimp.

The second time was in April of 1993 when I took psilocybin (hallucenogenic mushrooms) to accelerate my process by moving my assemblage point. (A Don Juan ploy). Only I had very little previous experience with it and took way too much. I never would wish a trip like that on anyone. It was so tremendously terrifying and exhausting. It lasted 12 hours. I had flashbacks frequently for months. Each time I relapsed, I went into a nauseating green no exit terror nightmare and I felt clutched by death.

The third time was in November 1994 in Chico, California when Kel and I were with Leonard on his property doing austerities, working our process and helping Leonard. Leonard was supporting us to move volumes of old karma and conditioning. I took advantage of the energy and took on too much to address from my programming.

The result was an incredible toxic release in my physiology. I had hives in every square inch of my being. Every orifice—inside and out had huge hives. I also manifested about 25 more symptoms. We moved into a motel because the perpetual itching disallowed me from wearing clothes, sleeping or eating. I was insane for a week from this. Kel was at his wit's end. It took me more than a month to eliminate all the toxicity.

The fourth time, of course was with the senility. I hope to shout that this is the last time I ask Source to empty me so mightily all at once. It does not have to be hard, to get excellent results. I have to constantly remind myself that the net gain will be well worth the journey.

When we believe in Life Everlasting, we have all the time in the world to accomplish our goals to manifest our dreams and our desires. In order to do this **we must take action continuously**. And we must be loving, gentle and compassionate with ourselves and our process as we do this. Affirm this for yourself, so it can become your habit.

If we procrastinate, become lax and develop a mañana attitude or we believe it is somebody else's job, we lose. With those sabotaging thought forms, we can never be recipient to the Glory that has been and is waiting for us.

23) DIFFERENT OPTIONS

People steeped in mortality and the inevitability of death have a difficult time understanding that there are other options. People steeped in unconsciousness who live their lives as if they were bullet proof immortals fare no better. It is imperative that humanity: 1) awaken to their lives and 2) to other possibilities besides death , because death is soon going to go the way of the dinosaurs.

There are those in body on the Earthplane that have been here for hundreds and thousands of years in the same body. These **Physical Immortalists** learned to master their body-mind. And there are yet others who have learned to be single minded. Because of their love for God, they have **translated** (transfigured) and now enjoy planet Earth from a much higher place than mere mortals.

I was fascinated by Baird Spalding's writings **The Teachings and Lives of Masters of The Far East.** I found his experiences awesome and was totally intrigued by his interactions with Jesus, Buddha and the precious folks who knew how to take their bodies with them wherever they chose to travel, no matter the distance...They came and went like the wind.

It didn't feel like Spalding got it. Maybe it was not his destiny. For me, the books fell short. How did those people have the understandings and grace to be able to share time with the Buddha and Jesus in being able to serve others the way that they did? How did they get to have their lives seem so effortless?

When I first read **Anna Lee Skarin**'s books, I really got jazzed. Anna Lee is a **translated being** who has come back to share the treasury of God's gifts. She tells us exactly how to do it. Anna Lee makes it sound so exquisitely simple. I am certain it is that simple…we just have to get out of the way.

Anna Lee Skarin was a Mormon who was banished from the Mormon Church as a result of her beliefs. So fearful of her were they, that they actually produced a body and a death certificate. God bless them. She pays them no mind, because she knows and lives the Truth of her being.

When a person decides to love God with all their might, the might of that love replicates itself in the subconscious, transmuting the miscreated experiences of lifetimes into the love of God. As the conscious decision to continue emptying the subconscious unfolds, the conscious and subconscious harmonize and eventually incorporate the superconscious. The result is that they become one mind—the person then becomes "single minded". I finally know what it means to be "single-minded unto the Lord".

And when a person learns to love God with all their heart, mind and soul, that love fills their being and purifies all the misqualified energy in their body mind into higher truth. When a person has sufficiently purified themselves, choosing God's Light rather than the sewer of their mind, they are born again in the sacred waters of the Spirit. Thus they are called twice born.

We have been in unbelief so strongly about our true beginnings and thus our true nature, that our hearts have become very hard. Our job now is to disbelief everything that we have believed with regard to Separation and open our hearts, bodies and minds to the real presence and support and love of God here now.

"As one perfects love within himself, the dross is burned away…This comprehension of the power of love and learning to send it thru the entire body is part of the divine method of OVERCOMING mortality with its sordid condition and grim penalties…The process of translation is done thought by thought, cell by cell, as one completely spiritualizes his entire being and becomes clothed in Light.

For 'Man can evolve from the man kingdom into the God Kingdom'."
(**Beyond Mortal Boundaries,** Anna Lee Skarin)

When a being achieves translation, they may choose to go into Union with God-Goddess or they may choose to continue on the Earthplane in service to humanity. They become like bodhisatvas—beings who complete all their karma, but choose to return to be in service to hasten the awakening of Humanity to their Divinity. Translated beings, however, have the ability to travel the earth in the blink of an eye.

Anna Lee reminds us that Jesus' teachings were not about death; they were about Life Everlasting. Yet by all appearances, it looks and feels like we are entrapped in the 3rd dimension, by our stuckness around the Crucifixion. It is as if we all gasped at that moment and have been stuck in a time warp ever since.

What then of the Resurrection? What do we do with this fabulous proof of translation? Is it so far removed from our windows of possibilities that we can only respond as a deaf, blind, mute? Jesus overcame death. He overcame it, because he thought he could. You can too. If you allow yourself the possibility.

Look. You know where you are now…what country, socio-economic level, governmental dictates you now are facing. How long has it taken you to get the understandings you have now about life—your life, about God—your God, about the Cosmos—your Cosmos? Do you want to give this all up and have to begin anew gathering yourself and your understandings?

Do you want to take the risk of being born in a much more challenging environment next time? Choose any one of a dozen—war and famine are increasing daily around the globe. Why not keep what you have and go further into wakefulness, wholeness and Union? It is Not more work than finding yourself in Uganda or Bosnia next time. Don't you remember? It is also not more work then finding yourself in a nursing home this lifetime either. Just think about it for a minute and them take action continuously.

I used to have a real aversion reading the Bible or anything that sounded like the Bible. I had a problem with <u>The Course in Miracles</u> in the early 1980's for that very reason. My right-wrong around religion forbade me appreciating scriptures of any kind for a long while. Reading Anna Lee, however, puts a completely different perspective on passages from the Bible, because God explains them thru her. Treat yourself to her books.

Physical Immortality does not mean that you maintain your body forever in a decrepid, degenerated, aged state. Physical Immortality is choosing life and not death in your every moment. As a result aliveness is your focus and your goal. More than anything **Physical Immortality is about improving the quality of your life right now**.

By consciously choosing to be physically immortal in the now, you do not fall victim to deathist thought and living; you are not under the continuous sabotage of the death urge and death. Consciously choosing and taking action in Physical Immortality is the best face-lift you can give yourself; it is the decision to youth.

By choosing Physical Immortality, you get to prove your Union with God-Goddess—which is your natural state. Physical Immortality was given to us in the Beginning. Reclaim it as a continuous choice until it supercedes your separatist conditioning and supports you being more awake to your life, to your habits, decisions and actions.

Why would one want to choose physical immortality? Why would anyone want to stay on earth indefinitely? Many immortalists have said because the Earth is such an interesting place. More than that, I would add that this is a gorgeous planet. Mom is really beautiful and I want the opportunity to experience that beauty again and again. Boredom is not in my experience.

My friend **Leonard Orr** became interested in Physical Immortality 40 years ago. He began reading immortalist philosophy and then discovered that all the authors were dead. So, he decided to seek out true immortalists—people who are Living Immortalists, not just people talking about it. People had to be over 300 years of age to qualify as an immortalist for Leonard. He found eight such folks and he knows there are many more.

One immortal goes to the forest one day a week to do fire (sit with fire) for a 24 hour period to purify his body-mind. Leonard asked another (who allowed people to only come as close as 150 feet to his person), what he attributed his longevity to. The gentleman replied, "Stay away from people".

Bhartriji or Bhartrihari as he has been called throughout the ages, lives in Sariska National Forest in Rajastan, India. He has resided there for well over 2000 years. As a matter of fact, he precedes Christ's Earthwalk. (He told Leonard that he and Jesus had the same teacher—Babaji of Hairakhan).

On Bhartiji's property are 7 tombs dedicated to his past deaths. Yes, every 108 years, he kills his body. It is laid to rest and entombed in concrete. Within a short time, he recreates another body. Bhartriji has freed himself of Samsara (bondage in the unending cycles of mundane existence thru death and rebirth). The next time he will demonstrate his mastery over his body will be in 2006. Kel and I plan to be there.

Bhartriji calls himself a yogi and not a guru. He does not see himself as a teacher for others. He sees himself instead as a devotee to God. His service is to God. Even though he is not as available as many gurus are, if you call him he will come if your intention is pure.

Bhartiji was a noted scholar, grammarian and poet in varying centuries. At age 300, he wrote a Satakam (100 verses). The following is one of the verses of the **Vairagya Satakam**/Refuge in the Forest:

"The cyclic recurrence of sunset and dawn
Daily serves to measure life's decay.
Man does not grasp time's fugitive flight.
Seeing old age, pain and death
He is not aroused to anxiety.
Drunk on delusion's heady wine,
The world is mad in oblivion."

He says he was not enlightened when he wrote it; he says he did not get enlightened until he reached 700 years of age. This Satakam is a satire and is the only nonbuddhist document that buddhist monks must copy and learn as they train to become monks. Copying or reading the Satakam can change your state if you are in a funk or an upset. (To read Bhartriji's fascinating story, order your copy from Inspiration University).

Babaji of Hairakhan is perhaps the most phenomenal immortal that Leonard (and others of my teachers have) met in person. Babaji is not only an immortal, he is also a Mahavatar, which means he does not come thru a woman's body as avatars (beings who have realized their God consciousness such as Jesus, Satya Sai Baba, Amma Chi, Mother Meera, etc.) do.

He usually builds a body with consciousness. He says it is a lot of work to do this. Babaji has mastery over his body even when he is processing the sludge of the world. He is capable of having more than 13 bodies at any one time on Earth.

Babaji is a reincarnation of Shiva, that aspect of Deity whose job it is to destroy Maya-darkness-illusion-Separation from the mind of man. Babaji comes to the earthplane when there is need. His job is to remove the veils of deception from our body-mind.

Babaji is the "Angel of the Lord" in the Bible. To me, He is also Mother-Father God. He is the Goddess and reminds us to be in adoration of the Feminine Divine within. He is supporting all of Humanity in healing their Will essence on this Will polarity Planet. Baba is the inspiration in my life and I am incredibly grateful.

Babaji used to bathe at 3am and 3pm everyday in the Ganga River. One time when Leonard was assisting Baba, Leonard thought to himself "I wonder how old this body is"? Babaji said to him, "Very old body". Leonard not missing a beat, asked "How old"? Babaji said "Over 9000 years".

You can learn more about Babaji of Hairakhan by ordering books, cassettes or videos from Leonard at Inspiration University or either of the Babaji ashrams in the U.S.: Haidakhandi Peace Center, Rt.1, Box 60, Malmo, Nebraska 68040, **www.babaji.net** or Haidakhandi Universal Ashram, P.O. Box 9, Crestone, Colorado 81131.

What Leonard learned from spending time with these immortals is that they held one common denominator or success formula. They attributed their body-mind mastery to the use of Spiritual Purification. Spiritual Purification is using the elements of Earth, Air, Water, Fire and the Ethers to purify the body-mind and our environments of polluting thought-feeling-energy.

Spiritual Purification consists of doing simple, delicious basic practices on a daily basis which cleans and maintains our energy body-mind. Spiritual Purification practices are the perfect anti-oxidant for our inner and outer environs. They support youthing and joyfulness in our lives. See next chapter.

Besides being aware of the above options, it is also important to recognize how the aging process is at work unconsciously in our world. It is conditioning—from our family traditions that will be replicated unless we intervene.

We generally memorize the aging process by watching how our parents, grandparents and other relations did it. So whenever your Mom and Dad started looking old, is probably when you will put into practice that learning. Your mind will decide when to do it and your body will obey. This is generally the way it works—the body follows the dictates of the mind...unless of course you intercede with Higher Thought and practice and countermand the conditioned learning.

You can start right now this very moment by releasing agedness, decrepidness, degeneration, death urge, death wish and suicide from your body-mind. You can also release senility and infancy consciousness (which go hand in hand when you are in the process of senility).

You can also release your old conditioned fear and terror of aging, dying, senility, etc. There is a ton more you can release if you think about it. And if you cannot come up with what to release, find an excellent Rebirther or Q.D. Teacher or call or email me (505-382-

8771; toni@anextstep.org) or Leonard (540-885-0551; rebirth@rica.net).

Another great thing you can do for yourself is to start celebrating yourself daily by thinking of yourself and referring to yourself as an eternally young being. Allow your new signature in life to be preceded by the adjective "Young"…as in Young Toni Delgado. See what an incredible leading edge that puts you in as you lead yourself and others into delicious Everlasting Life…Heaven on Earth In This Body Now. (Thanks Leonard).

24) SPIRITUAL PURIFICATION PART I

✦

"The Wise Do Spiritual Practices"

Spiritual purification is all about cleansing our energy bodies (to include the electromagnetic field or aura) with delicious practices. These practices are ancient ways of honoring the energy body—our sacred trust. Adopting these practices into our lives assures us of good health, well being, longevity and Union with Source.

These ancient ways are called Sanatana Dharma—the Eternal Religion belonging to all humanity regardless of creed. Sanatana Dharma strengthens our spiritual and higher purpose here as an endless reminder that we are ONE, eternally connected to Spirit, each other and the Cosmos.

Spiritual Purification (or the practice of Sanatana Dharma) is a habit that promotes awareness and clarity. It caretakes and cleanses our energy bodies quicker than most other practices. When you do spiritual purification, you are working with the elements of earth, air, water, fire and the ethers. There are many ways to work with the elements. We will list a few and encourage you to creatively develop your own.

The beauty of working with the elements to purify your body-mind-field is that they are so exquisitely simple. Using them cleans you faster than your mind can clean you. You don't have to do anything except remember to participate with them. That's all! It doesn't get any easier than this.

Water:

1.) Shower or bathe at least two times per day. Washing off the accumulated pollution from your process and others' will enliven you, refresh you and extend your life. Leonard Orr (founder of the exquisite healing tool called Rebirthing or Conscious Energy Breathing) says that indoor plumbing has been the primary factor for people living longer today.

2.) Drink ample clean (reverse osmosis, spring or distilled—not tap) water every day. This will keep your internal fluids flowing and support your colon function. (If you don't have an elimination for every meal you eat daily—you are constipated. Drinking more water and especially taking Dr. Richard Schulze's herbs at—1-800-herb doc—will help). Drink up to 64 oz of good water every day depending on your size.

3.) Do wet rebirths—consciously breathe in a bath tub or hot tub with a trained facilitator till you learn to do this on your own. Contact us: toni@anextstep.org or Rebirth International—1-540-885-0551.

4.) To introduce more energy into your clean drinking water, put a clean crystal, semiprecious or precious stone into a sun tea container or glass jar. Let it sit over night or in the sunlight. When you drink it, you will be getting the benefit of both the pure water and the healing energy of the particular stone you have chosen. (For cleaning stones contact us).

Air:

1.) Get conscious with your breath and how it relates to your body-mind health. Contact A Next Step…light center for emotional healing toni@anexctstep.org or Inspiration University distributor of Leonard

Orr's books. PO Box 1026, Staunton, Va. 24402. We recommend: Breath Awareness and The Healing Manual. Gay Hendricks in his book Conscious Breathing also has excellent exercises.

2.) Find a Rebirther—a breathing facilitator—who still is consciously breathing themselves on a regular basis. (Call Rebirth International for list—1-540-885-0551 or email us for an appointment: toni@anextstep.org). Do ten to twenty sessions or more. Commit at least to ten sessions to learn how to do it yourself and how to support others in going through a full breath session.

3.) Take time to be with Mother Nature. Sit in fresh out of doors air with the sun behind you—twenty minutes is good or longer. Take time also to walk gently, slowly, consciously with relaxed full inhalations and exhalations. The desert, parks, forest, beach, waterfalls are grand places to do air purification with your sacred breath. Walking slowly on Mother Earth also helps us learn patience.

4.) Working with any form of pranayama will purify you, discipline you (the discipline will raise your self esteem) and make you happy. Rebirthing is an excellent form of pranayama (breath and vital air control).

Earth:

1.) Working with color is a great way to use earth energy to support you. While learning colorology isn't imperative, it is helpful. Otherwise, use your intuition for the color that best balances you in the moment. This includes color of clothing and accessories, your living and working environment, the color of foods and liquids you ingest. Color also can be introduced into your meditation and healing work.

As with all energies, colors have high and low aspects. Here are some examples: Red—power, enlivening, raises body temperature and blood pressure. Orange—power color, good at reducing pain. Yellow—promotes flow of creativity and our constitution, great color for inspiring your creative writing. Green—increases energy, proliferation of energy and abundance. Blue—calms, soothes, lowers body temperature and blood pressure. Pink—confidence booster, great to wear when publicly speaking. Turquoise—enlivens spirit, great to wear when feeling depressed.

2.) Working consciously with food is using Earth purification. You can learn to become sentient enough to eat foods that your body tells you it needs to balance your energy. (The tools taught at **http:// www.anextstep.org** can and will raise your level of sensitivity to become aware of your bodies'desires instead of old habits.) Eat fresh and raw fruits and vegetables often. Learn about juicing. Use fresh foods as medicine to create glorious health and life extension. (Check out N. W. Walker's book <u>Fresh Vegetable and Fruit Juices).</u>

3.) Using herbs internally (in teas, tinctures and Dr. Schulze's intestinal formula 1&2 and Superfood) and externally (in baths, poultices, salves and balms) is an awesome way to consciously work with Earth energies. Many herbs in stores are radiated (this kills and poisons all vital energies). Grow and/or harvest your own or find out the sources you can get your organic herbs from. (Dr. Schulze's people have excellent information. Yes, we like him. And Sam Biser's Save Your Life Video collection on Dr Schulze and others is excellent: 1-877-485-5004)

Dr. Richard Schulze is the king of pure herbs. He was a student of the late Dr. John Christopher and Dr. Bernard Jensen. Dr. Schulze knows there are no incurable dis-eases or situations of the body. He has taken people through every dis-ease you can think of, with herbs and other strategies (ie. hydrotherapy and more). The colon is where all dis-ease and death begin. Clean out your colon with Dr. Schulze's incredible formulas—he even tells you how to make them. Call 1-800-herb doc (437-2362), to get free information.

Fire:

1.) If you have a fire place or a wood burning stove, you are indeed fortunate to have a living flame available to you within your shelter. Use it to purify your environment and your energy body. Sleep with/

near fire if you can. The only fire better than the above is an open fire outdoors—there is no restriction of the flame and energy. It is an efficient purifier of your energy body. All you need do is be within five feet to achieve maximum results. The fire can also clean your mind very quickly. If you are in a funk or an upset, the fire will burn away the heavy, uncomfortable feelings and change them to peace. There are several ways to do fire depending on your intention:

a) You may use fire simply as a purifier—a means of cleaning/healing you. Be willing to sit with the fire at least two hours or more or sleep with it. You will be shifted in temperament.

b) You may use the fire as support to your process in resolving long held grievances. You may wish to write the grievances down, throw them into the fire for release. Old letters and memorabilia—attachments to the past can also be burned and released this way. We have used the fire to rescind and release all karma from the past...marriages, divorces, relationships. We have burned wedding dresses with clients who remarried themselves to the True Self....Mother Father God.

c) You may build a conscious fire as the mouth of God—Goddess. Into the mouth of God, you may offer prayers of gratitude and petitions for support. Along with the prayers you may offer flowers, fresh fruits or vegetables, rice, nuts, popcorn, dried fruits or beans. A coconut is a good way to begin this ceremony and is an auspicious way to offer prayer for the planet, Collective and yourself (one coconut may be passed to all participants placing their opening prayer into this sacred seed or several coconuts may be used). Do not put trash or paper into this fire. This is a very simple sacred ceremony which you can add other rituals or traditions to. To learn more about this, contact us.

2.) If a fire indoors or outdoors is not possible, use candles. Get twelve candles. Light one and feel your body. If you feel nothing, light another and feel your body. At some point along the way, you will notice how many candles are needed to be the most effective in cleaning your energy body. Sit or sleep with this number. This practice is particularly efficient when we are in a healing crisis. Tall glass candles are great for this. You can usually find them in the Mexican section of your foodstore or in religious article stores.

3.) Having a lit candle in a working environment calms the energies that be. I frequently had a lit candle in my high school classroom where I taught, as well as in my counseling and massage office.

4.) Fire walking is an incredible experience. It teaches us to pay 100% attention to what we are doing and really stretches our windows. Our limitations and old conditioned habits of thought and fears get shifted whether we walk or observe others as they walk.

Ethers:

1.) Working with or using smudge sticks (dried sage tied and blended sometimes with cedar, lavender and other herbs) purifies our field and any environment indoors and outdoors. It is a habit we can adopt to use daily. It will absolutely support a cleaner environment and therefore healthier space. Intent the cleaning and purification of yourself and your space. Light the stick. Use a sea shell under it to prevent burning of carpets, furniture, clothing, etc. It is the sacred smoke that purifies us.

2.) Using incense is another way of working with the etheric energies. It can calm, soothe and provide sacred space wherever you are. Some incenses seem to have higher vibration than others. We have found Nag Champa (a favorite of Satya Sai Baba) and Shivranjani (a favorite of Mahavatar Babaji of Haidakhand) to be highly beneficial.

3.) Intent is involved with ether energies. If you are living and seeking your highest desire, then you are utilizing the high aspect of the Ethers. If you are enmeshed in slug consciousness, you are involved in the low aspect of Ether energy. Where are you in your consciousness and life? Are you awake? Do you know your highest desire?

You will often be able to blend the use of the five elements into your ceremonies,rituals, prayers, pathwork, japa (repeating a name of God) and daily activities. We find spiritual purification to be easy, fun and pleasurable. We especially enjoy these techniques when we are purifying our minds and bodies using the specific tools we use and teach.

One of the most beautiful and powerful ways to incorporate all five elements is in the Sweat Lodge. Each Native American Tribe has its own way of doing the lodge and the purification of sweating. It is good to learn and participate with several different traditions to honor the sacredness of this experience.

You however, may come from another tribe—your own. Create your own sacred way of doing a Lodge and Sweat. For us, the Sweat Lodge is a living being, a gift from Wankan Tanka and Earth Mother. It can transcend right and wrong. The Sweat Lodge offers us a way to profoundly connect with our true essence and the elements that we are.

25) SPIRITUAL PURIFICATION PART II

◆

"The Wise Do Spiritual Purification"

You are a sacred living temple. Mother Father God reside in every cell of your being.

Everything that you do for yourself to caretake and maintain your body mind, you do for God. God-Goddess are sacred guests within your dwelling. The kindnesses and intelligent choices you make with regard to diet, exercise, emotional release work, mental health, relaxation, career, relationships affect your living temple and therefore, your relationship to Source. Following are suggestions for further Spiritual Purification.

MIND—Mental Body

Your mind does not reside within your cranium. It exists within all that you are, your body and field. It is an awesome part of your being. It is not, however, the most important part as it would like you to believe. The mind thinks it knows everything, but it does not. It contains a lot of information. And quite a bit of that information from our physical experience is inaccurate. It contains old conditioning—acquired programs that are generational and our reaction responses to life which are learned perceptions.

Much thought in our physical mind (and particularly the subconscious) is sabotaging. The opportunity we have here is to become conscious of these patterns and learn to reframe them. Taking no action with our mental processes allows the mind free reign of our energies. This exhausts us. We are mostly not aware of the drain that our mind puts on our system.

The mind plays all day long and all night long. Some people call it "the monkey mind", others call it "the chatter box" or " the committee". Some people are not aware of it—they have become numb to it. Some people are driven crazy by it. Our opportunity with our mind is to improve the quality of our thought and thus the quality of our energy and lives.

Some ways to address what is held in your mind are 1) the Twenty Connected Breaths and the Basic Thought Meditation. 2) Getting Rebirthed—learning to breath energy as well as air. Rebirthing releases held tension in the body which is caused by our thoughts—feelings. Find a good breathing coach who still rebirths themselves. Do ten—twenty sessions with them and more. Then learn to do it for yourself. Contact: Rebirth International or A Next Step…3) Learn Quantum Dynamics which attends to both our mental and emotional bodies. It transmutes (chemically changes) matter into Light and Energy…purifying…energizing. It allows us to let go of upsets in ten seconds or less. Contact : A Next Step…4) Working with affirmations is good, but slow if you aren't releasing the tension of the thoughts and feelings creating them. The previous strategies work well to address this tension.

FEELINGS—EMOTIONS—Emotional Body

Every single thought we have in our body—mind has one or more emotions attached to it. For example: the thought "I am not enough", could have attached to it the feelings—emotions of sadness, resentment and self abasement. Our emotional body is the largest of all of our bodies—composing about eighty percent of who we are. We have within our body-mind a huge backlog of suppressed feelings—emotions. We have suppressed this information for a long time, mostly because we have learned from our culture that this expression of ourselves is wrong. We have lots of opportunity to embrace, acknowledge and revibrate this aspect of self…our emotional body.

The Twenty Connected Breaths with the Basic Thought Meditation are good ways to begin purging the emotional body. Rebirthing, Reiki, BEST chiropractic, massage and Quantum Dynamics are excellent tools for this. Body Electronics (point holding) is another remarkable tool that can change the emotional body and one's physiology as well. Any emotional releasing tool you feel comfortable with will serve you. Understanding and mastering your emotional body is paramount to Spiritual Purification and successful living. You cannot become enlightened until you have evolved yourself through your emotional issues. And…you cannot heal if you cannot feel.

SACRED SOUND

Mantra is sanscrit for the sacredness of divinity presented in and through the vibration of sound. Mantra is the name of God spoken aloud, creating a healing vibration within your body. This sound frequency reverberates through your being calling God-Goddess present into your physical reality. Continuously repeating a mantra or name of God is called Japa. There is great merit in doing Japa on a mala.

A mala is made up of a varying number of beads—depending upon the particular culture or tradition. In India they use the number 108. A hundred and eight beads is the sacred number. The number was arrived at by multiplying the 12 astrological houses by 9 planets.

While malas are made up of different types of beads, stone (both precious and non-precious) and sacred seeds, it is the Rudraksha mala that is said to bequeath the greatest merit to wear and use. The Rudraksha bead is called Shiva's Tears. It is said that Shiva did an open eye meditation for a thousand years. When he completed the meditation and blinked, he shed a tear, which became the rudrasha seed. The Rosary came from the mala; Babaji of Haidakhand was one of Jesus' teachers.

Mantras can be repeated in any language. However, be aware that your native language may have all kinds unconscious hotspots for you. Therefore, using sanscrit, an ancient mother language, may be outside of your consciousness enough to have more impact spiritually on your psyche and thus be more healing. Sanscrit is a language sacred to this planet.

Here are some suggested mantras:

OM NAMAH SHIVAYA is the Maha Mantra (great mantra). It can translate to " I surrender to God-Goddess", "Lord Thy will be done", "Infinite Being, Infinite Intelligence, Infinite Manifestation", "Truth, Simplicity and Love".

OM MANI PADME HUM translates to "Jewel of the Lotus" and is in reference to the Buddha.

Listening to or repeating out loud with such mantras as the Gayatri and Mahamrityunjaya is incredibly healing. Listening to bhajans or Tibetan chanting is also remarkably calming to our nervous system. Reading aloud or listening to sacred scripture is also extraordinarily healing. Deepak Chopra's Sacred Sounds—Healing Verses volume one and volume two are highly recommended.

Toning sound has become a healing art that many practitioners are employing for themselves and others. Working with 13 different tones can heal most ills of the body.

The Kung of the Kalahari would encircle a member with a fractured bone, tone for them and the injured person would immediately be healed.

Some folks doing this work know that toning sound creates a deeper connection to Higher Power. Here are the names of some of those using toning for healing: Mark Patterson at godiswithin@excite.com (beautiful CD-Angels Caressing You), Tom Kenyon, Jonathan Goldman, Wayne Perry, Sherry Edwards, Gina Solat, and Daniel Konkel.

SACRED SCRIPTURE: *Written word*

These texts may also be read aloud or silently and listened to; both mediums bring merit for the participants as well as healing. Suggestions: The Puranas, The Mahabharata, the Bhagavagita, the Ramayana, The Course in Miracles, the Bible, the books of the Essenes, the Koran, the Talmud, the Kabbala; any written work that inspires one to be closer to Source.... the list could be very long.

All books of the lives of saints, immortals and avatars; Autobiography of a Yogi, All books about Babaji of Haidakhan, Satya Sai Baba, Ammachi, Mother Meera, Goraknath, Bhartriji (or Bartrihari). All books about physical immortality by Analee Skarin, Leonard Orr. We receive a boost to our immune system reading the words of an empowered guru or author. Truth—Divine Truth purifies and nourishes our bodies—minds.

SACRED SYMBOLS-*Tatwas-Yantra Yoga*

Tatwas utilizing elements of the earth create a visual healing vibration for our bodies and our environment. They reflect the Divinity that we are. Reiki, Quantum Dynamics, The Light Bridge Attunement utilize symbols as part of their healing vibration. They are keys to consciousness and enlightenment. The Light Body Ascension Chart, a tool used by Quantum Dynamic Practitioners has the tatwas of the seven fold chakra system in addition to having 9 systems of healing the chakras. (Contact us at A Next Step to order your own exquisite Light Body Ascension Chart toni@anextstep.org)

LOVE

It is important that love be included in the gift of Sanatana Dharma—Spiritual Purification. Without it, we are empty like Shel Silverstein's Missing Piece...seeking to fill ourselves with everything but us. We wander without direction. Love is a guide- post for us. It is also an integral part of our being that we have armoured ourselves against.

God-Goddess has consistently told me these past ten years, "Do only what you love. Eat only what you love. Buy only what you love. Live only where you love. Go only where you love". So…find a job or career that satisfies you and brings you joy. Do what you love—no excuses!

Decide and then create a loving relationship with God. It makes no difference what you call God. What matters is that you do it. You are never alone anyhow. Once you commit to this relationship, you will "get" that **you have support all the time.** Talk to God. Eventually you will "get" Their communication to you. This is your primary relationship.

Decide to have a loving relationship with your body-mind. Treat your body like the sacred loving temple it is. Nurture it, bathe it, loofa it , massage it. Make intelligent choices in what you feed yourself and what you drink. Choose to be more conscious, to eat live foods. Exercise—even if it's just a walk around the block or jumping on a trampoline or have someone jump on a trampoline near you. This loving focus on yourself is highly purifying. This is your secondary relationship.

Decide and then create loving relationships that can support you in your process called life. Once you've made the commitment to have a loving relationship—first with God and then yourself, you will find it easier to do this with other people. This hierarchy and order of intent with God first, yourself second and others third, creates perfect balance in loving relationships.

Balancing giving and receiving is sometimes difficult for people to surrender to. The Circle of Life is both giving And receiving. Many of us are prolific at giving, but really shy in the receiving department. Be willing to ask for what you desire, then be willing to graciously accept it with gratitude and ease.

The intent of love creates light, aliveness, vibrancy and vitality. It youths and energizes us. ALLOW LOVE TO BE THE MOTIVATION OF YOUR LIFE.

FORGIVENESS

We must address forgiveness as we speak of love and Spiritual Purification. There will come a time when forgiveness will no longer be a necessary requisite for healing, because we will be beyond the need for forgiveness—we will have nothing to forgive. Indeed there will even come a time when we will be beyond healing and the need for it. Until then, we have a lot of old conditioning to get thru to find that doorway.

Because misunderstanding, judgement, blame and guilt have formulated so much of our Earthwalk, we have a backlog of lifetimes of relationships and experiences to forgive. Sometimes we become so traumatized by hurt and pain, that we find it difficult if not impossible to forgive others and especially to forgive ourselves. AND...forgive we must.

Staying stuck in unforgiveness creates tremendous hardness in our hearts, minds and bodies. This kind of stubborness creates a bitterness that toxifies our outlook on life. Every relationship we have...with people, money, food, etc. gets infected with it. Eventually it will kill us.

So please hear this and take it in, "**YOU HAVE NEVER, EVER DONE ANYTHING WRONG AND UNTIL YOU GET THIS, YOU ARE BLAMING SOMEONE, SOMETHING OR YOURSELF AND NOTHING CAN HEAL**".

Be willing to at least begin forgiving. Pray and allow Source to support you in getting through all that you felt and believed with each experience; acknowledge it, transmute it and love it free from your body-mind—each and every hurtful situation.

Also recognize that while you may wish to be at total forgiveness, you can't rush it. Any attempt to control and force it, will prolong it.

Be willing to trust the process. Go with it, for as long as it takes. It has its own timetable. Ask for God's Light in Patience.

26) THE BREATH OF LIFE

In Genesis 2:7 of the Bible is written "And the Lord, God formed man of dust and breathed into his nostrils the breath of life, and man became a living soul". In Ezekiel 37:5 is written " Thus saith the Lord God unto these bones: Behold I will cause breath to enter into you, and ye shall live".

And so it is that the Lord God has caused us to live thru the breath of life. We take this gift of life and the breath that sustains it so for granted. It is not even a thought we have; we are so busy with our "doings".

We are alive and kept alive at the insistence of our breath…and it behooves us to learn more about the anatomical features of our breath, its physiology and what significance and opportunity this gift creates for us. Better said: everything within us is energy and the energy of our body-mind is very much affected by our unconscious patterns/habits of breathing in a defended body-mind. Did you know that your breath can move and change your energy?

Conscious focused breathing can change our physiology and thus our reality. It can change our emotional state. It can change our mental frame of mind. It can relax and calm us, allowing us to be at ease and more at choice with our creations. Our coping skills get greatly developed. We can then focus, center, balance and create with more awareness.

To demonstrate this, take a minute to check your breathing pattern right now. Notice how small or large your breath is, how shallow or deep each breath is. Notice how your body feels. Can you feel your body—and not with your outside hands!

Our opportunity is to learn about the energy of breath within us and then learn how to use this energy to its maximum efficiency. What follows are significant and important methods of pranayama (sanscrit for breath control) that can change your life forever to the better.

26 A) TWENTY CONNECTED BREATHS

This exquisitely simple breath technique will ground and center you in a couple of minutes. You will be using a connected breath, which means you will be connecting the inhale to the exhale without pausing.

Use your fingers to count as you breathe.

You will be doing 4 (four) short inhalations and exhalations. Then 1 (one) long inhalation and exhalation which equals 5 (five) breaths or 1 (one) set.

You will do 4 (four) sets of these, which equal (20) twenty connected breaths.

Resume your normal breathing when you finish. You will notice that your (normal) breath has expanded and that you feel relaxed and good. Some of you may feel tingling or a bit light headed. This will pass as you continue with your normal breathing pattern.

Do this breathing technique only once a day for a week before you go on to the next breathing exercise. However, if you have been a student of pranayama, you may continue on to the next exercise immediately.

26 B) BASIC THOUGHT MEDITATION

This technique could also be called Emotional Upset Release because it effectively moves both thoughts and emotions. Every thought we have, has one or more emotions attached to it. In essence we have emotional thoughts.

Example: Thought—I am rejected.

            Emotion—(this rejection) causes me to feel pain, self pity and grief.

This thought and these emotions (emotional thoughts) cause us upsets.

Here is what to do with each upset.

1) <u>Define the upset</u> : **"The thing I dislike or hate the most about my life right now is**_____ **"**

Feel your body. Do the twenty connected breaths. Feel your body again.

2) Be willing to <u>go to neutral</u> . Even if it feels like a lie, do it anyway. Your subconscious does not know the difference between what you think and feel, what is real or not. It will always go with what you say.

"It is okay that the thing I dislike or hate the most about my life right now is_____ **".**

Feel your body. Do the twenty connected breaths. Feel your body again.

3) <u>Gratitude Statement</u> Gives you the lesson of this process. Open to receive it; even if it is just teaching you that you <u>can</u> move the energy of the thought-feeling.

"I am grateful that the thing I dislike or hate the most about my life right now is_____

because_____ **".** The "because" is "the gift; the lesson".

Feel your body. Do twenty connected breaths. Feel your body again.

You may feel light headed or dizzy or incomplete. Just continue with a connected breath; balance will come shortly.

You also may not feel much in your body. We have been shut down and disconnected for a long time. Don't worry, you will begin to feel as you persist and continue using this exercise.

27) CONSCIOUS ENERGY BREATHING (REBIRTHING)

People say that the most dangerous thing on the Earth is man. My belief is that the reason he is the most dangerous is because of old conditioning. It is kept alive in our body-mind—in our emotional thought which manifests into action, creating our reality. Our conditioning in large part, is unloving and full of misunderstanding. Our conditioned emotional thoughts are fraught with danger. They stop our energy and ultimately, they kill us and sometimes they kill things and other people.

In order to return to the love that is—the love we are, we must be willing to find this conditioning within us and change it. We cannot do this with our mind alone. As Satprem says "You cannot heal the circle with the energy of the circle".

We must find and align with greater powers within us to champion our minds and change this conditioning. The sacred breath is such an ally. In order to love yourself enough to keep yourself from harm, you must spend time with the Sacred Breath of life within you.

It will help you empty the conditioned emotional thoughts—the baggage from lifetimes past. What could be more natural than allowing the Breath of Life to support you into Heaven on Earth, into Life Everlasting, into a higher quality of living now?

The famous japanese filmmaker Kurasawa once said, " It is impossible for a human being to talk about himself with any honesty". We are habituated into lying and most of us have no clue that we do this. It is a part of our defendedness against the world we perceive as dangerous. It is a shield we use. And by and large, it is an unconscious shield.

Our internal dialogue is what maintains our belief system and our reality. If we choose to change that dialogue, our reality changes and so does our conditioning. The words we use to keep this dialogue in motion maintain the chatter. Most of what we tell ourselves is a pack of lies that either we decided or took from someone else as truth.

The Hawaiian and other native tribal peoples had awareness long ago that our mouths are the purveyors of dishonesty. So when it came to creating beautiful sound with their magical flutes, they did not use their mouths with which to do this. They used instead their sacred breath. They create their music thru nose flutes.

The sacred breath that is used in Conscious Energy Breathing helps us empty the habit of this dishonesty. It purifies our body-mind. It purges us from the tyranny of our old conditioning by changing and upgrading the quality of our thought. We get reprieve from the ceaseless mind chatter also. We get to see and experience life from an enlightened point of view. Our body-mind drops its white knuckle death grip, we relax and are given a different, more supportive way to believe and do things. It is as though we are given new eyes with which to proceed.

New neural pathways are grooved in our brains, as old ruts get filled up with Light, Love and Understanding. Blame and guilt, old conditioned fear, terror, paranoia, suppressed and repressed anger, hatred, resentment and rage get acknowledged, forgiven, transmuted with the power of the breath and loved free within you.

I was intrigued by the idea of Rebirthing when I first heard about. It took me several months to garner the courage to do my first session (July, 1980). I laugh now as I look back at the experiences and all the reflections that were given to me that I could not appreciate fully at the time. My ego was too big and I was "dumb", as Don Juan would have said.

No matter all the ridiculous stupid self talk, my Higher Self was directing me, thank goodness!...So, I continued. My second year of rebirthing, I found an excellent psychotherapist who used Rebirthing as her therapeutic strategy. (I had asked Spirit for both a good woman psychotherapist and a good woman Rebirther). Thank you Goddess for the thousands of multiple healings I received from You thru Gigi Delaney. God bless you Gigi wherever you are.

In those breathing sessions with Gigi, I pulled out the cork of long held stubborn stuckness and began my really serious journey into healing...into starting to learn about who I was...into seeing who my parents and grandparents were as people and not just taken for granted biological family. I was able to understand a little of why I am here. I was able to understand some about my fears and anger. I started taking responsibility for probably the first time in my life for my life. And I started to get to know about the God within.

I am grateful for all the work I did with Gigi and most of all I am grateful that I allowed myself to surrender enough to recognize and know that love is real and can be trusted. It was from Gigi that I learned about unconditional love and started learning how to lovingly detach.

It was Gigi and a few other rebirthers in those early rebirthing years, that told me how fortunate I was to have manifested rheumatoid arthritis. I thought they were absolutely crazy. I had no idea at that time how **contentment can breed stuckness, decay and stupidity.**

I was raised to believe that safety and security (which I learned I absolutely "needed") were achieved in keeping life as stable and changeless as possible. So my white knuckle death grip was well in place at an early age. I maintained that posture til my body-mind could not handle that grip any longer.

Breathing those first several years was like picking up an incredibly old dirty, wrinkled throw rug that had never been shaken or cleaned; shaking it out real good and then throwing it into a washing machine. Those first years of rebirthing opened the door to the grandest adventure of my life. I found out I was holding on. I found out I could let go—at least begin letting go. I could forgive—at least begin forgiving.

Being able to heal matters generationally was incredible to me. I was able to see/feel/change patterns that I carried from my mom, grandmother, father and grandfather and on back. It was even wilder to be able to reframe those old conditioned tapes from past lives.

It was an incredible purification process that I began. I had a lot to purify. We all have a lot to release; we're holding volumes...literally lifetimes of muck. And it is why we are here...to release this debris. We will not have to revisit every lifetime. Our Higher Power will bring forth those most relevant; those that give higher understanding to unravel the lies.

Being able to go back to inter-uterine memories to feel myself, my parents and our tapes was a rush. It is amazing how consciousness is with us at conception and before. And it is amazing the decisions we make (made other lifetimes) and remake that are founded in misperception and misunderstanding. The awesome thing is being able to change all those miscreated experiences into wisdom and good.

Conscious Energy Breathing supports us thru the power of the breath to not only access these memories, but also purify and reframe that which we thought-believed-felt was true into Higher Understanding.

The energy of the matter of our mind is mostly heavy. Holding it, withholding it, suppressing it, hiding it, hiding from it takes an incredible amount of energy. Which is why we feel so heavy and fatigued. Immune deficiency dysfunctions and other dis-eases continue to escalate in this country for this very reason.

We don't even have a clue of how energized, light and healthy we could be and feel until we start and continue to Rebirth. The breath lets go this suppressed material and all the tension we are applying to it, to keep it controlled and at bay.

When we learn to breathe energy as well as air, we learn that the energy we get from consciously breathing, supports us in feeling lighter, happier and healthier. Our life force (Chi, Ki, Prana) gets a boost and we want more of it with which to do life.

As the body-mind let go of what it has been holding, a variety of sensations are experienced (ie itching, cold, heat, burning, pain, etc.). Everything our body does is perfection because **Our Body Does Not Know How To Do Anything Wrong**. It just does what it is told from our programs—conditioned memories that have been stored in our subconscious mind.

Leonard called this system of breathing "**Rebirthing**" at first, because he discovered how excellent it was for releasing birth trauma and creating a renewed experience of life for the body-mind. Our breathing gets shut down from the arduous birthing process. It's not only our Mothers who work hard to deliver us, we work incredibly hard to maintain ourselves in perhaps the hugest paradox of life: being born feels like certain death.

Most of us do not consciously recall our births, but our bodies remember the hellacious experience. The birth—all we thought-felt-perceived gets imprinted into our psyches, creating a template that we will replay again and again in all of our relationships, lifetime after life-time, til we consciously relive this experience to free ourselves from it and reframe it. In Rebirthing we gain this freedom. We also free our breathing mechanism thru the breath release.

In the ancient Vedas and Purana texts of India, over and over the sages and rishis talk about doing the correct rituals, ceremonies, pen-ance, sadhanas necessary to get off the wheel of karma; to be free of the need to reincarnate; to be free of the need to come thru the womb of woman.

Leonard says, while the birth trauma is a necessary point of address, it is infancy that weighs even heavier on our development and health. Infancy consciousness is a highly frustrating period of helplessness, hopelessness. While we are bustling with life force energy, we feel and are incapable of doing anything for ourselves. We are totally dependent on our caregivers. And even with the most loving, attentive caregivers, infancy is a drag. It lasts a lot longer than the wretched birth process.

With every perceived negative that we take in, we shut down our breathing apparatus even more. Sometimes all of life feels traumatic when we are wet, hungry or in pain with colic or gas. And this process of shut down continues as we grow into the process of life and face all of our reflections.

Feel your body around learning to crawl and walk. Around falling down and hurting your body and pride. Around potty training and all those times you missed. Feel your body around being afraid and no one coming in to see about you or hold you. Feel your body around kindergarten, elementary, jr high and sr high school. Feel your body around college, grad school. Feel your body around exams. Feel your body around peer group, dating, fitting in and feeling insecure any way, feeling like a nerd and not belonging. Feel your body around all your uncertainties of sex and your sexuality.

Some of you won't be able to feel anything around these issues, because you are shut down and not connected to your body from the multiple traumas of life. This is not wrong or right. It just is. You shut down a long time ago to protect yourself from feeling—feeling anything; for you felt uncomfortable and unsafe back then.

Now you must allow yourself to begin feelng more and more to heal your true nature, so it can fully come back into you. You cannot heal your unconscious belief in separation if you do not allow yourself to feel everything you felt and believed about how separation got created for you. **It Will Not Be As Painful As You Think It Was.**

The Sacred Breath will wash away all the muck of all life trauma, purifying your body-mind-soul of all perceived hurts, injustices, wrongful judgements, misunderstandings. You will shine and be radiant with a renewed vision of life—your precious life. God Understanding and Wisdom will fill your being with the most outstanding grace, joy and supreme satisfaction.

Rebirthing or Conscious Energy Breathing can be learned in about 10 to 20 sessions, depending on your karma and process. It is highly recommended that you learn and breathe with a rebirther/breathing coach who breathes and processes themselves regularly—at least once a week, not once a year. The One Year Seminar is a great way to both learn how to breathe yourself and others, and also a great way to create spiritual community which is sorely needed all over the planet.

The One Year Seminar is made up of a group of people committed to their process who are willing to support others and receive support thru the gift of Rebirthing. It meets for a whole day once a month and once a week for support. You can contact Rebirth International (RBI) for information on One Year Seminars across the globe and you can contact us for One Year's in Southern New Mexico. Leonard also offers the OYS experience via mail. The people in the One Year Seminar in southern New Mexico also incorporate the gift of Quantum Dynamics which accelerates our individual and group experience. (RBI email **rebirth@rica.net**; A Next Step…email   toni@anextstep.org).

28) QUANTUM DYNAMICS

Physical Immortality is the gift of life that Mother-Father God breathed into us at Creation. God gave Everlasting Life and all that They had and all the qualities that They were to us, their children. We were given the finest existence—the most quality life. Yet, how many of us feel, know and remember this? We are so disconnected from our Divine Beginning that this inheritance feels like an impossible dream. We have become so emotionally dead that our spiritual essence has become a sought after avocation instead of a prized absolute.

In order now to retrieve this Eternal Gift of Life, we must invest time and energy to undo the falsehoods we have learned to subscribe to that pull us toward certain death. Undoing these lies requires addressing our body-minds' conditioned and suppressed emotional thoughts. It means taking this energy (because that's all we are—energy) and revibrating it into the truth consciousness of our Union and Divinity.

Our fear, stuffed anger, hateful resentments, blame, guilt etc. yield low frequency energy which work to sabotage us daily in all ways—physically, emotionally, mentally and spiritually. When we seek to admit, acknowledge and address these emotional thoughts with tools like Quantum Dynamics, we become less dense and we become more conscious and awake. This changes how we think, feel and who we are. It offers us more choices.

Like Physical Immortality, Ascension is also a change of consciousness. We in essence ascend within ourselves; evolving the human experience into the God experience which we can have in these bodies now. As you work thru your low frequency into higher frequency, you melt away the lies of separation and become One with your true spirit and the spirit of everyone else. This merging into The One Energy is called

God. Q.D. is a magnificent tool to assist us into Physical Immortality, Ascension and Godhood.

Quantum Dynamics is working with the elements of fire, air, and the power of the spoken word within us in an incredibly easy and peaceable way. Quantum Dynamics is a tool that allows us to let go of upsets in 10 seconds or less. What it actually does is it **transmutes** (alchemically changes) the **density** (the accumulated emotional thoughts and experiences that make up our conditioning within our being) **into Energy and Light**.

Quantum Dynamics laser beams our focus (whether we hold it in consciousness or not)—a thought-decision-judgement-belief-opinion-misunderstanding—and changes it from matter/mass into Light and Energy. It addresses feelings-emotions by revibrating them into higher frequencies of Energy, Light and Love.

It allows suppressed and repressed material to be accessed from the subconscious and gives you an easy, efficient way of handling it. (It is so simple that your controlling ego may not get its grace and dispensatory gift at first). With it, you can recapitulate and transmute all upset and conflict back to Origin, when you are ready.

Q.D. is excellent at transmuting conditioned programming into Light and Energy, shifting baggage (psychological debris) into aliveness. As such, it is an exceptional tool for those folks serious about quality living and especially Physical Immortality and Ascension into their Godhood. In order for us to achieve these lofty states of being, it is necessary to address all parts of self including the shadow.

The shadow holds aspects of self that most of us deny or hide. People will say "I don't even want to go there". But go there we must. All must be known to lead us to authenticity and honesty—truth. Looking at the shadow feels dangerous and warlike to folks. That's why many avoid it. If we are to heal war in physical reality, we must be willing to heal it from within first.

War, in outer reality, feels incredibly infantile and naïve to me. I don't feel like it creates solutions. Mostly, I think it is an incredibly devious, corrupt and manipulative ploy. Most wars are economic power games with high price tags that countries play with each other. Language differences exacerbate the power relationships that create war. People don't fare well communicating in the same language in a given culture. We fare even worse cross culturally. Words fail us even when we speak the same language. As the book of Murdad says "Words are at best an honest lie".

Couple the above with the fact that most adult looking bodies are emotionally wearing diapers. Heads of state, heads of companies—corporate America—, heads of families and all the folks underneath the heads are baby thoughts encarcerated in large bodies. This planet needs for its people to get thru their infancy consciousness, so they can become responsible, emotionally mature adults.

Most of us have not been schooled however, in the rudiments of the emotional process. We don't even have a vocabulary to talk about what we might be feeling. Rebirthing helps a bunch and Quantum Dynamics teaches us emotional literacy. Q.D. gives us a vocabulary with which to express ourselves. Having the words to talk about what's going on gives us confidence, wisdom and the freedom to express what formerly we had no words for. It also gives us permission to get into our feelings and emotions without judgement, shame or penalty.

Having this ability to transmute previously huge, avoided/denied issues into immediate Energy, Love and Light increases our self esteem and self worth exponentially. We get lighter and lighter, wiser and more aware fast and easy. It helps us get thru infancy consciousness, power relationships and a myriad of other conditions of the human experience quickly.

Of all the tools I use, **Q.D. speeds the increase of conscious awareness and perception** in an individual faster than any other technology I have ever worked with. It is efficient, practical, fun and easy. It connects us to God-Goddess (or however you choose to relate to your superconscious) so we are never without support.

Q.D. is an incredible way of undoing stuck patterns of being, dysfunction and dis-ease. It is a tremendous boon in this crazy world filled with chaos, overload and full tilt change. It will teach you to accelerate your path of learning and healing in a gentle and harmonious way.

Q.D takes the accumulation of conditioned ways of being and stuckness generationally and from other lifetimes and compresses them immediately into the present moment of now, releasing them and replacing them with higher and superconscious decisions and understandings.

It connects you to your will, your emotional body as you have never been connected before. And creates within you a personal power you have not remembered for a long time—perhaps for millenia. It teaches you to honor and express your will without judgement as in the past. With Q.D., you become a skillful observer and participant of your process.

Q.D. allows you to be habitually at choice, because you know what to do in every moment, as you allow yourself to be supported by the simple strategies of Q.D. Your emotions no longer use you; you learn to use them to advantage.

Q.D. is so practical, everyone can use it. It creates self responsibility, ease of communication and ability to end all conflict and war from the inside out. With Q.D.,.the concept of reflection is much easier to accept. If you don't like what you see/feel in the reflection, you can change it at its core—within yourself.

With Q.D., we learn to release blame, wrongful judgement and all the stuckness of that conditioning. We learn about the components of our control drama, about our addictions, attachments, white knuckle death grip, self abasing self talk and other destructive habits of the shadow. All of these behaviors and thought–decisions can be released and replaced by higher and superconscious thought and habit.

We learn that old conditioned resentment, hatred, anger and rage are emotions that must be acknowledged, so that they no longer rob us of well being and vital life force.

We have such fear of them that we avoid, deny and suppress them which is a habit that stops our energy, creating ill health and unhappiness for us. Q.D. allows us to change these habits now.

What folks don't realize is that most times we have the elements of blame, guilt, fault, hurt, kill and revenge attached to the above emotions. It is these latter components that are decisions or below body death emotions that feel awful...and they can be released.

When we release blame, fault, hurt, kill and revenge out of any emotion, we are able to experience that emotion in its pure state. We can then take that emotion and raise its frequency—its life force (our life force) to a much higher frequency of Light, Love and Energy. This strengthens our will—our free will and supports us in becoming more sentient, conscious and aware. We also become more courageous and fearless.

Q.D. helps us keep our heads above the constant sea of change and the barrage of information that we are continuously exposed to day and night—it is in the airwaves. People live in perpetual overload; they operate (sometimes poorly) in struggle, most of the time and have little consciousness about the "soup of confusion" they live in. Q.D. can change this situation tremendously. It can give clarity, simplification and ease as folks release this 7th chakra conditioning.

Fear seems to be a huge part of the Collective consciousness right now and has been for a while. Periodically, the fear rises to terror (9-11-01) and then bounces back and forth between fear and terror. As a result of feeling trapped in fear and terror and our fear and terror of them, we also feel paranoia around our creations. We can absolutely revibrate the emotions of fear and terror and release the paranoia with Q.D.

Championing our emotions and our suppressed emotional responses of the past allows the "driver of our bus/our head of state" to be a mature, level headed adult, rather than a cranky, fearful child or an angry, rebellious teenager. Championing our emotions does not mean that you suppress, deny or restrict them in any way. It means we can now face them and any situation fearlessly, acknowledging them and breathing them into higher frequency Energy with the Q.D. attunement.

Many people's experiences with Q.D. is that as they work their way thru old anger, fear and resentments, etc., they find themselves emptying...so that what formerly triggered them into blaming rage, no longer has that same effect. Many people are calmer, more serene as they own their reflections and work with them.

Quantum Dynamics gets activated within us thru an attunement that is given. It utilizes sanscrit symbols and shakti energy. The attunement creates a battery pack of power within us to address everything that comes up with confidence and ease. Calling on this battery pack, we are hugely supported to joyfully release the conditioning of misqualified energy out of our subconscious and out of our body-mind. We use the power of the spoken word and the sacred breath to activate the battery pack within us.

Q.D. came into my life 4 months after I was told to change my lifestyle or I would be a goner. Two months after I received the attunement, I was sitting in my bedroom at 2 am with my suitcases packed, ready to leave for an American Massage Therapy Association national convention. I was also supposed to start teaching the fall semester that same week. As per usual, my plate was overflowing.

"What was I doing?", I thought. My young adult life had been dedicated to hard work to make a difference and to receive recognition for my efforts. As a mexican-american female, I prided myself at being able to participate in undoing the stereotype of lazy mexican in America. I was driven by my controlling ego.

That nite in my bedroom, I felt torn between my different worlds, my priorities and the words I had received from Spirit thru Ram Dass months earlier. I lay down to rest for a few hours, before I had to leave for the airport.

I dropped off to sleep and dreamed that God came before me to inform me that I was at a crossroads. I had to make a choice—the path of Light—Spirit or the path of darkness—ego. I woke up at 3 or 4 am clear with my decision. I was done with the need for approval from others. I quit all my offices with the AMTA nationally and statewide. I now chose to dedicate myself to my spiritual unfoldment.

I am certain I would not have been able to let go of my addiction and attachment to receiving recognition and getting approval from others, if it had not been for Q.D. It made the choice/change easy. Q.D. not only changed my life, it probably saved my life. It has changed my life in a big way multiple times now. It instilled in me a confidence and a knowing about my connection to All That Is. I am so grateful to Mother Father God for this powerful, gentle, easy technology. This remarkable tool continues to evolve.

29) INNER CHARACTERS-
GATHERING THE SELF

Part of our process is that who we are is a compilation of a cast of characters—every age, size and sex within. Each of these inner characters is holding different parts of the puzzle. Most of them want address. Some are very wounded and untrusting and not willing to come forth right away. And they must be addressed in order for us to become whole again. If you are willing to be there for them, then you can have a relationship with them.

You may ask yourself, "How did all these aspects of self come into being?" The answer is that we have been fragmenting since Origin. Every lifetime, when we chose to die, we fragmented. And each lifetime, when we experience trauma or perceived trauma, we fragment.

Our opportunity is to gather our parts. We can do this with our willingness to work with our inner characters and with competent facilitators and excellent tools like Rebirthing, Quantum Dynamics Process, Hypnotherapy paired with Q.D., Body Electronics, etc.

As you work with your inner characters, you heal that fragmentation or denied part of self. This is an inner guidance system of soul retrieval. It is a way to become whole and Holy again. As your inner characters and the issues they are holding are addressed, they can take on new job descriptions that you and they design for themselves. These new job descriptions allow healthier thought forms and ways of being for them and you. Those that are wounded children can mature as they heal and grow with you.

You will also encounter very evolved, divine beings within, who have been waiting for you to awaken to their presence. They become awesome allies for you and your process. They also are great advocates in working with your cast of inner characters. Sometimes, when your inner characters feel completed in their process, they choose to go into Union with Mother Father God. When they go into Union, more of you will also go into Union with the Divine.

When you have gathered yourself and developed enough personal power within, you will be able to gather the parts of yourself that exist outside of your body. Mother Father God call this your "lost will". (Ceanne DeRohan Will Books) Your lost will fragmented from you at Origin. You must develop enough personal power from gathering yourself and committing to your assignment here in order to become whole and holy unto yourself.

30) TOUCH

Touch is a very essential ingredient of life that many of us are missing as Ashley Montague reminds us in his exquisite book <u>Touching</u>. Again, because of our learned habit of impersonalness (due to our disconnect), we have little connection to our bodies (and indeed other people's bodies) in any healthful way. There are a variety of ways to learn to reconnect to your body healthfully that involve touch.

Touch is a phenomena that cannot be over stated. "The greatest sense in our body is our touch sense. It is probably the chief sense in the processes of sleeping and waking; it gives us our knowledge of depth on thickness and form; we feel, we love and hate, are touchy and are touched, through the touch corpuscles (nerve endings) of the skin". J. Lionel Taylor, <u>The Stages of Human Life</u>, 192, p.157.

We all long to be touched,—yes, even those who claim they do not want to be touched…they too long to be touched. "Tactile experience is as basic as breathing, eating, or resting, in that without its satisfaction, the organism cannot survive". Ashley Montague, <u>Touching, The Human Significance of the Skin</u>, 1971.

Some folks are afraid to touch others and afraid to be touched—they learned to be afraid. Some learned it isn't "proper" to touch. Some remember that touch is dangerous because of this life or past life abuse. Still others believe affectionate touch (hugs) lead to sex. And I am certain there a lot of other thoughts around touch that have not been mentioned here.

We are sentient beings. We were created to be sentient. Sentient means feeling. Feeling has to do with touch. To be healthy and whole, it is our nature to be connected to our bodies. Touch is an excellent way to help us reconnect, heal and become whole again.

It is easy for us to pick up and touch babies. It is difficult to hug and touch people as they age. We love babies, and we have a phobia around the elderly. It's like we are afraid we're going to get the old age they have.

My ex-husband's grandmother became increasingly withdrawn and senile when she was put in the nursing home after she lost her husband. She started not recognizing family and friends who came to visit and their visits became fewer and fewer. She always knew when I came though, because I was the only one who touched her. I made certain I held her and touched her every time I went to see her. I guess when we truly disconnect from our bodies and our realities, we lose touch with reality in all ways.

The eldery need touch just as badly as the newborn. In the throes of senility, Kelley's touch as he did B.E.S.T., massage and Reiki on me helped anchor my body to my Spirit as I drifted in and out of consciousness. It is as if his touch loved me into being when I felt almost as though I was not.

There are a variety of ways to reconnect to your body healthfully. B.E.S T. chiropractic, Massage and Reiki are a few ways that can support you in reconnecting to your body. They will also create marvelous healing for you as well.

30 A) B.E.S.T. (BIO-ENERGETIC SYNCHRONIZATION TECHNIQUE) BY DR. KELLEY ELKINS

B.E.S.T. is short for Bio-Energetic-Synchronization-Technique. B.E.S.T. was developed and is taught by Dr. Ted Morter D.C. of Rogers, Arkansas. I was fortunate enough to have been in the charter class at Parker College of Chiropractic, Dallas, Texas in 1982 when Dr. Morter was the president of the college. When we started, there weren't but about 32 students and not a lot for the college staff to do...compared to several semesters later. Dr. Morter would, on occasion, take the last few minutes of a class and entertain us into the next class with his view on chiropractic and healing. I thought and still do, that Dr. Morter is genius.

I entered Chiropractic college at 34 years young with some questions. I wanted to know why a patient had to repeatedly be "adjusted" or have the joint(s) physically manipulated again and again? Why couldn't they stay after the "adjustment" where they were designed to be? Dr. Morter answered those questions.

I also learned a lot in VietNam. I had the good sense to learn everything I could while in the service. I was a veterinary technician and often I was the veterinarian, while stationed with the 595 military police sentry dogs in Danang and Quang Tri, Viet Nam. There I started questioning among other things, the systematic antibiotic therapy that I had been taught to administer to those dogs in need.

One afternoon in Quang Tri, a handler brought a dog in, that under normal circumstances, would have received antibiotic therapies. However, something snapped in my brain and I told the handler he did not have to walk the ammo dump that night. I told him to put the dog back in its kennel and return to the clinic. I told him I wanted to "keep the dog under observation". I had no idea what I was doing.

The handler returned and we talked about "stuff". Then I asked him what was going on with him. He replied either that he had received a "dear john" letter or one of his parents was ill or getting a divorce…something like that. When I asked him how long he had to go "in country", he replied it was only a month or two or less. I said, "Well then, why are you so worried about the "problem", when there is nothing you can do about it here…put it on the back burner until you get home".

The handler with a sigh said,"Doc, you're right, I'm being foolish " or something to that effect. We both looked at the door, as we heard his dog bark signalling to us that the dog was fine.. I asked him to bring his dog back into the clinic. He asked if he was going to have to walk that night. I said "No, you're off tonight". He brought his dog in and the dog was normal to every degree. I was amazed at what I had just learned. **The dog was doing the handler's problem.**

So, when I entered class at Parker, I was looking for what was causing the body to dysfunction. Why are we calling everything an accident or certainly someone else's fault? Dr. Morter taught us that the body cannot do anything wrong. It doesn't know how. He told us that the body is listening to the subconscious mind. The subconscious mind is never wrong, just not always appropriate.

I learned through Dr. Morter, that the largest organ of the body is the skin and it is also the most sensitive. Through appropriate touch, the body has to respond in a way that can absolutely change all matter of symptoms and causes. The subconscious mind is that part of the mind that is in charge of running the body. Consciously we don't have time to know what every one of the 75 to 150 trillion cells are doing, much less the various organs. And they are not on automatic pilot.

The subconscious mind knows exactly what every cell is doing and doesn't judge it as right or wrong. So, consider this: when we are angry, every cell of our body is angry…when we are happy…every cell of our body is happy. This is truth. Science has proven it, especially as a result of the wonderful research of Dr. Candace Pert PhD.

Through the capacity to ask the body what to do and where to do it, the body like a computer, has to upgrade. All systems, organic or non-organic, given the opportunity to return to their natural state will do it…every time.

Let me give one example of how wonderful B.E.S.T. is. We have all known or heard of people that have lost a limb or hand or foot. They complain of "phantom itch" and/or "phantom pain". This phenomena can best be explained in this way. If we took all the appliances of any household and plugged them all into a single wall outlet and turned them all on, the electrical system would "throw" a breaker switch to prevent an electrical fire.

This safety mechanism is excellent. And the human body works the same way in reverse. If there is a significant amount of neurons firing toward the brain mixed with fear and especially terror, the brain will also "throw" breaker switches. Consequently, for the amputee, there are parts of the brain that never learned that the limb is gone or that anything happened at all.

There is no way to know how many breaker switches the human body has. We do know that the breaker switches can be "thrown" before we are born. If our mother believed she was about to be injured physically, mentally or emotionally, not only might she have "thrown" breaker switches; so would we—residing in her womb.

Here is an example of what I am speaking of. While working on a male client some years ago, I was simply holding points about his head, while he relaxed on his back on a table. His left leg kicked up and out so hard, I thought he was going to lose his lace up shoe. Bringing his leg back, he asked me what I had done to his ankle. I replied that I had done nothing, what had he done? He said "Nothing, I'm just lying here". I asked him to go back in time, what had happened to that ankle? He replied that was impossible. I asked what happened? He said, "Twenty five years ago that ankle had caught an AK-47 round in Viet Nam". I told him, "Well, your mind just found out about it".

The mind/brain is a delicate organ. Science knows so very little about it. Medicine claims that with anesthetics, there will be no pain. This is correct. However, breaker switches will be thrown and the healing of the surgery may never really complete until the mind/brain knows there is something to heal. Furthermore, if the mind/brain knew in proper time that there was need for surgery and given the appropriate touch and herbs, the surgery would probably not have been necessary. I say this because this has been my experience time and time again.

I will admit though, that this is not always the case. I held my stepfather in my arms as he pleaded with " I want out", I glanced at my mother and his eldest daughter. I then calmly said," Then go, man". He died in my arms. His dis-ease and diagnosis of pancreatic cancer had been robbing him of life too many months before he would allow me to work with him.

His death urge was stronger than his life urge, having been debilitated so thoroughly by the cancer and the horror of chemotherapy. We did, however, for the first time ever have the most awesome conversations on everything including death. I didn't know how much I loved him and I am grateful we got to heal our relationship with the gift of B.E.S.T. as the facilitator. It allowed him to have a much more peaceful passage to his next place.

Let me repeat: **ALL SYSTEMS GIVEN THE OPPORTUNITY TO RETURN TO THEIR NATURAL STATE, WILL DO SO...PROVIDED THAT THE BODY-MIND WANTS TO.**

30 B) REIKI

Reiki is an healing ray of light that brings to the Earthplane Universal Life Force Energy. It is an incredibly beautiful gift of love that has been given to us. Reiki exquisitely expresses Babaji's teachings of Truth, Simplicity and Love.

Mikao Usui brought forth the activation of these ancient symbols. He searched high and low for them for a long time. It is his lineage of Reiki that Hawayo Takata brought to the Western world. Gratefully it continues today to grace the world and our lives.

Reiki is about love. Love is about Union—ONENESS. Reiki helps us become whole unto ourselves as it releases obstruction—blockage in our bodies. Sometimes it triggers memory of past lives as it releases.

Reiki creates a slowing down, a catching up with ourselves. It creates calm, peace and serenity in the middle of our often full and chaotic lives. It offers a relaxation that we can create in minutes. And it is only in the quiet of relaxation, that we can truly find our"selves" and heal.

I love that it is a foolproof system of healing. You can't do it wrong. Wherever you place your hands, the Higher Power of yourself or who-ever you have your hands or intention on, sends the perfect amount of energy wherever it is needed. The same is true if you send it long dis-tance. We aren't in charge of the session…God-Goddess is.

God uses the energy in the most efficient manner, taking it to the right place, in the right amount. And it happens quickly. For this rea-son, Reiki is a great way for us as healers to learn to completely get out of the way with our ridiculous controlling egos and learn that all heal-ing comes from God. We are merely the instrument.

There are only two contra-indications for Reiki and they are contra-indicated because Reiki does work so fast. Do not do Reiki 1) directly over a severed appendage, til its been put in its right place or 2) directly over a fracture, until the bone has been put in its right place. Once the appendage has been sewn back on or the bone set, then you can do

Reiki over the area of duress. While waiting, you can do Reiki over the rest of the body to calm the person or yourself.

The first couple of years of senility, I gave myself Reiki everyday, sometimes all day long because pain was such a constant. Reiki reduced the pain in my pelvis, legs and back.. I also had stabbing pains in my eyes and head which Reiki moved. I used Reiki to help me move emotional energy pollution after being with groups of people as well.

I give great thanks to God for the healing ray of Reiki. It is so simple, it should be in everybody's body. We can be using it everyday to help us out of confusion, insecurity, tension, pain, discomfort, feeling helpless, hopeless, etc.

Children can give it to themselves, each other, other members of their family, including pets. Adults would find it helping them all day long on themselves and those in their lives. Reiki teaches both humility and responsibility. It teaches us that not only do we all matter, we are all sacred.

30 C) MASSAGE

Massage is thought of by many as a luxury. For me, it is a necessity. It is a wholesome, healthful way to maintain a balanced circulation. It lubricates and exercises all the systems of the body—like a good workout, but without the fatigue. It supports the release of toxins thru the avenues of elimination, encouraging healthier skin, lungs, colon, kidneys, liver, etc. It also promotes an incredible sense of well being. As it helps us relax and let go the tensions of the day, it calms and nourishes us.

In addition to the purgative and calming effects of massage, it also addresses the largest organ of the body—the skin. The skin is a huge doorway to our sentiency and vehicle to get us to connect to our bodies and "selves". It can support us in memory retrieval, allowing access to suppressed trauma. Massage creates an excellent opportunity to release conditioning that locks us into the past, which left untapped could create illness and dis-ease.

When my massage clients and friends started getting triggered on the massage table during their sessions with me, I saw the grace that came from pulling Q.D. into the session. This is when Spirit started showing me the gift of pairing these tools together. Shortly, thereafter, Babaji asked me to become a Q.D. teacher. Process Massage (massage and "head work") is what I called it when I moved to New Mexico.

I love massage and I love what it does for my body-mind in both health and undoing dis-ease. There are many varieties of massage techniques as well as varieties of massage therapists. We all have unique energies…see who suites you and your energy. A certified massage therapist may be what you are looking for. Know that not everyone with a piece of paper (credential) is going to guarantee that you're going to receive a good massage or a massage of value.

For me, "a massage of value", is a massage whose effects last a long time in my body.

Some massages feel good, but because the therapist's energy was not what it could be, the effect only lasted a few hours. I love it when a therapist is working their process on some level and the effect of their masage lasts in me for several days.

Shop around. Go to several different therapists. You may settle on one person. You may like trading off with several. I found out who was good in and with what. In Wisconsin, I went to six different massage therapists to suite my body-mind energy. Some were soft touch. Some worked me to the bone.

A hard, deep massage (deep tissue work) is not what you need to reconnect with your body-mind, with your "self". That type of massage will only promote you staying in numb. To reconnect to your "self", you require a soft touch, so you can learn to begin to feel.

31) OLD CONDITIONED FEAR OF RIGHT AND WRONG

With right and wrong being such a conditioned reaction-response, humanity in the main, fears making mistakes and fears feeling failure. We are so crystallized in these thought forms that people participate limitedly in life for fear of being made wrong or making themselves wrong, for fear of being criticized and condemned. These fears keep us postured in stuckness and contraction.

I have for the last several years told myself and clients that failure does not exist in nature and man is a part of nature. Consequently, all we are capable of is decision making, followed by action and learning. We are continuously engaged in learning from deciding/not deciding, from acting/not acting. This approach to life serves me well as I replace old conditioning with it.

And, I want to share with you a similar approach with the old conditioned languaging that I got from late nite TV. Charlie Rose was interviewing Robert Redford, Glenn Close and two young directors about the Sundance Art Community Project in Utah. It was a remarkable exchange and presentation.

Sundance is the brainchild of Redford. He put it together 30 years ago. It offers an incredibly suppportive community for artistic film expression replete with resources unavailable anywhere else. Artists, directors, and actors experiment in the Theater lab to create their vision—their creative expression (their essence of life).

Gregory Nava, the creator of both the movie <u>Mi Familia</u> and the weekly PBS-TV series "The American Family", got his liftoff when he created the film <u>El Norte</u> at Sundance and brought home best Foreign film and many other kudos for it.

At Sundance, artists are able to put into manifestation their passion in what one of the directors called "a heaven like atmosphere" surrounded by resources and artists to advise them: where they and their project are the sole focus. They called it the BEST college you can think of for what you want to do artistically. When you bog down in your creative process, you have the opportunity to change your approach and problem solve with others who are interested in your process.

In this atmosphere people are actually encouraged to fail. They believe that is the only way a person can learn. They said failure was an absolute necessity for the creative process and that it is an understood and nurtured part of the experience there at Sundance. In the theater lab, people are given the chance to make mistakes in an environment of feeling protected. They know they are safe there to do this. They are encouraged to take risks to promote diversity and authenticity. Their passion allows them to connect to creativity and their vision.

Glenn Close talked about the experience at Sundance being very much about process. She said there isn't anything that can't be resolved thru the creative process. She said "All we really have is the process…we can never predict where great joy and creativity happen…it happens at Sundance because those involved love the process".

They talked about having the courage to risk something different and how the world was better for it; that thru risk, diversity is kept alive; that that is about as satisfying an experience as you can have.

My passion was stirred listening to these folks who are following their desire and encouraging others to do the same, who are living their lives as fully as they can and who are providing a school of learning where others can catch the spark of aliveness and keep it going.

It feels great to know that Sundance and all those involved there, promote authenticity and genuineness, and love enough to encourage creative risk taking. Sundance folks, I applaud and celebrate you. Thank you!

We can't be afraid to live. We can't be afraid to learn. We must be willing to take healthy risks; to live with passion and compassion for the "self" and others. We must be willing to feel and be real. **LIFE IS THE PROCESS**. Love it! It's your process. When we let go of mistrust and relax into our bodies, our creativity flows thru. We can't be afraid of the outcome of our decisions and actions. We must create for ourselves our own Sundance in our bodies and in our homes. Do it!

Glenn Close also said "The Internet is not a better communication system; it is a place where we are getting more numb. We constantly have to be reminded of our humanity"…as a result of it and how we have been choosing to live our lives sequestered fom each other, afraid to feel, afraid to be real, afraid of failure and afraid of difference. I agree with her entirely. I could not have said it any better.

32) ABANDONING THE SELF

Get the idea of getting out of bed, going to the potty, wiping, flushing, going over to the wash basin, looking in the mirror, brushing your teeth, getting in the shower, and the cascade of activities that follow as you work your way up FULL TILT into the busyness and the doings of the day. Are you breathing in a way that will support the energy you will need to do this day well? Are you connected to your body or are you numb? Are you connected to God; have you brought God consciousness/awareness into your day (body) or do you (like most folks in the West) figure you have to go it alone?

Where is your center? Where is your balance in your day to day routine? If it is not created and sustained from within with Source thru your conscious decision, chances are your outer reality will reflect this to you—if you are awake enough to see it, get it, understand it.

Living unconnected—"unplugged"—everyone and everything for us is a convenience. We maintain impersonalness in our personas as a very important part of our control. Even in the sexiest, lustiest trysts, when we act with abandon in sex or lovemaking (both acts are the same; one has no attachment, one has attachment), we still hold ourselves back. It is part of our defense physiology; we built it in. We hold onto this because we think (consciously or unconsciously) that it is necessary for "the stability of our psyches". It is how we control ourselves emotionally, psychogically and physiologically; it is how "we pretend to feel safe and loved". (Thank you Bill Dempsey and Peggy Davenport).

Even in great relationships with a parent, grandparent, trusted friend, while we relish and cherish our precious moments with them, withholding energy happens on both sides. We withhold our energy—parts of ourself and we hold our breath to create that wall of protection/that wall of defense to hold it in place.

What is it about us that we can't trust ourselves or the other person enough to be fully present or true? Some of us say, "It's the other guy's fault". Some of us do 'fess up though. We just don't trust what appears to be love…what appears to be real. In fact the genuineness of real love terrifies some of us.

It's like we got slammed so hard, way back when that just in case we're right—that "it happened the way we think it did", we'll hold back so we don't have to crumble from the inside again. It's hard to live feeling like you're in a totally caved in, crushed state. It hurts to breathe.

Not trusting love and not believing that we are love creates a perpetual unconscious state of self abandonment. We abandon ourselves to a far lesser god…other relationships, our jobs as breadwinner, bill payer, caretaker, running here, running there…never quite out of struggle in our daily, ordinary, unplugged lives.

If we behave that way day to day, what do we do when the bigger challenges—explosions happen? Because they will happen. They can't not happen with so much denial of our true nature. We think that the way things are is natural, normal. We couldn't be further away from the truth. Explosions happen when our bodies, lives can't handle the pressure that has been building from living out of synch with our nature. Our bodies beg us to take notice…to wake up…to do something.

Heart attacks, strokes, cancer, AIDS, HIV are examples of explosions. Earthquakes, tornados, hurricanes, volcanic eruptions are examples of explosions. Remember, we are the Earth—we are not separate from the planet we live on.

How many of us say, "Oh, that will never happen to me" or "That kind of disaster will never happen where I live." How many of us bury our heads, so we don't have to think about or feel our running way from ourselves?

What about the myriad of minor explosions that we disregard as unimportant? Dr. Arthur P. Guyton, M.D., in the most studied text by medical students, <u>The Textbook of</u> <u>Medical Physiology</u>, says that "99% of all sensory input is disregarded by the human brain as unimportant". Good God! It is a miracle that mankind has been able to pull off civilization as far as it has come! We have because we are so loved and supported, and because we have a lot of help that is not visible to the human eye.

Every single event in our lives comes as reflection from our unconscious emotional thoughts conditioned by lifetimes of repetition. Yet, so few of us say to ourselves, "What about this has to do with me?" Very few of us have the awareness, the courage to take that reflection and do something with it within ourselves, so we can alter the recording and change the conditioning for good.

Every plugged up toilet, every sore throat in us, every illness in our children or our pets, every dead car battery, every sprain and broken bone, every "forgotten" deed is a reflection of some goings on in our programs, in our conditioned emotional thought process.

Every argument, every anger, every fear, every guilt, every feeling expressed in our presence has something to do with us or we wouldn't be there witnessing it. Somebody else would be there instead getting an opportunity to see a part of themselves...to take that energy message to learn from...to own it...to breathe with it...to move it and translate it into Energy and Light.

How many of us take ownership of our reflections? How many of us blame who or what we see as something other than us? How many of us abandon the reflection and thus abandon ourselves?

How many of us, when the going gets rough; when we feel ourselves entrapped in the abyss of our emotions, completely "puddle" and act like we never learned anything about new thought. We act like all the teachings we got from all the seminars we went to, all the trainings, all the great books of instruction (the "how to be unbelievably happy" books we read), all the hours of enlightenment spent with our gurus, never happened. It's like we go into deeper amnesia.

We abandon ourselves in these upsets because, the conditioning of our programs is so formidable and because we have not trained enough to not abandon ourselves yet. **Nobody can abandon us. We can only abandon ourselves**.

Self abandonment is a 5th Chakra isssue. To process it, process self rejection, revenge, feeling unworthy to receive God's love, blame and guilt, feeling like you don't matter,etc.

33) REFLECTION

"The world is but a mirror for us to learn from". Can you even begin to count all the places you have heard or read this idea before? Do you believe it? Does it feel like truth to you? Does it feel like a blessing or a curse? Are you grateful or angry about it? Your reaction-response says a lot to you about where you are on your path. Be willing to look at your reaction-response.

I do not even recall the first time this idea was presented to me. I do know that I have been inundated with it for at least the last 20 of my 54 young years. So, I would imagine you have been too. It's cause Source wants us to become self empowered and the only way to do this is to be willing to take responsibility for our lives and these sacred living temples we live in.

As I write this in my backyard next to a delicious fire that is burning off the muck of my own process and the EEP from doing community, I reflect on all the attachments I am working to release. I want to become a "hollow bone" as Frank Foolscrow (holy man from the Ogalala Sioux) talked about to Tom Mail's in the excellent book <u>The Power and the Wisdom</u>. I desire to empty myself so totally, that the only reflections I can create are of genuine love and loving detachment. I have more work to do in this arena.

As stubborn as I am, I see a lot of humanity being equally stubborn; holding on to the past and not having a clue of their true nature, their Seed of Greatness. And I feel, it's not all my reflection, because I have understanding and acceptance most of the time. Sometimes, however, I just want to shake them and say "Hey! Wake up!"

I know stubborness is not all bad. My friend Tari Benvenuti has gotten incredible boons from her stubborness. She wrote to Babaji when he was still in Haidakhan, India, requesting permission to go visit him. He denied her request because she was "bursting with child". She went anyway. When he first saw her, he yelled to her "Hey Bambina,. What you doing here? Go home!" And her getting there, allowed her stay for a few weeks. Baba gave her the name "Tari".

It feels to me, however, that the combination of stubborness and angry attachment to being right is a deadly combination. I would venture to say that it is this combination that is probably responsible for lots of explosions in our lives.

This deadly combination is born out of fear. It manifests in rigidity of sameness, unwillingness to change, stuckness and huge denial. In this combination, all thinking is contracted and highly positioned. The inability to own this fear consciously creates blame, criticism, harsh judgement, rejection, loathing and abuse.

The more people buy into this fear, the more out of hand it gets and the more it controls them. When this fear goes mad, it is born into hatred. Hatred is what creates war—race wars, religious wars, political wars, etc. It is the poisoned belief that difference is wrong, evil and dangerous.

War is all about hating and killing the shadow—that part of self that is completely and totally rejected—to the point of revenge and annhilation. In war, we point our weapons of destruction at our own self hatred. Killing our "enemy", is completely rejecting, killing the reflection of self.

Vengeful rage and rejection of self hatred, creates the terrorist within us that so many of us are seeing outpictured right now in the wake of 9-11-'01. We are equally unwilling as a population to own the reflection of terror thus far.

When are we going to get that destruction of others is destruction of self?! There is no evil; there is only the small self—impotent, timid and fearful. We hate this about ourselves. We foolishly believe we can kill this outside of ourselves. Our focus is totally misplaced; denial is huge is this domain. We cannot kill this outside of ourselves, because

THERE IS NOTHING OUTSIDE OF US! It is our reflections that need address desperately now.

We are in a severe global humanitarian crisis—war, dis-ease, genocide, poverty, starvation, inhumane behavior, disempowered masses, corrupt governments, abuses and terrorism of every shape and size. The only way to end this insanity is for us to wake up and change what has been.

We must be willing to own our fears, our hatred, our anger, our terror, our rage. We must be willing to make friends with our will—our emotional body—our reaction responses to our creations. We must not be in habitual severe avoidance, criticism or judgement of our emotional expression or that of others.

If you want to stop suicide bombers from destroying themselves and others, be willing to address the suicide bombers within yourself. Acknowledge them. Talk to them. Cry with them. Enroll them into your genuine intent to heal yourself from all the darkness within. Get them to see that killing their bodies is destroying the sacred living temple of God.

We must be willing to own every reflection as a valuable opportunity. Every word and action that is taken in our presence is about us, if it triggers us in any way. And even if it does not trigger us (many of us are too numb to know), we have opportunity to own everything as a lesson for us.

The idea of reflection is a huge concept. It takes a while to understand it. It takes longer to implement it for true value. And Start! Be willing to own everything you see and hear as you. Ask yourself,"What about this has to do with me?" Process the thoughts and emotions you get into Energy and Light. Get lighter and lighter til all of your shadow is golden.

When your shadow is translated into its golden gifts, your attitudes will be of self love, self acceptance, self confidence, self knowing. You will be expanded, open, willing, grateful and highly creative. Your sense of life and sense of purpose to humanity and yourself will be celebratory and generous. You will embrace all differences in yourself and others as wholesome, good and part of the ONE. And you will see your reflections as beautiful, wise teachings.

34) HIGHER TOOLS FOR UNDERSTANDING

As you begin and continue emptying your psychological debris, the muck from your subconscious, "the island of the tonal" as Don Juan calls it, you get lighter and lighter. You are given clarity, confidence, a prepondrance of "ahas" and "hits" from Source about what to do next in your process. Your inner guidance system and you intuition expand by leaps and bounds, as you align with your Higher Power and take immediate action.

As you reach this place, you can ask for more tools and more support. If you doubt or are slow to follow thru, the information given you slows down and will come with less frequency. Release all self doubt and unworthiness to receive. Listen and take action. Once you take action, the ball keeps rolling in your favor.

There is all kinds of channeling happening now and lot of psychic opening. Many, believing they are separate from Source, feel they have no way of getting info with regard to what is happening in their lives or what to do next. They feel they do not have the gifts (psychic ability, intuitive) of others or the gifts others profess to have.

The psychic astral plane got created at the time of our fall (disconnect) from Source. The psychic-astral plane is filled with disembodied entities who sustain themselves on the energies of anyone willing to listen or pay attention to them. They profess to be learned scholars, sages, teachers and aspects of Divinity. They are not. They are psychic vampires.

Those entities from the psychic astral plane use people who use you and your energy.

Get into your personal power and demand to know who it is you are working with. When you get into your personal power, entities of the psychic-astral plane will not mess with you. They will not be able to deceive you, because you will be your own person. Your ability to discern will greatly increase as you free yourself from your old programming and become your own authority. They prey on the weak, gullible and disempowered.

As you empty your inner misqualified energy, you will get to a place where you will be able to connect directly to the energy of your Higher Power, to God-Goddess. You will get your guidance directly from Them. The communications will be clear and untainted.

One way of getting to that space and receiving high quality support is a tool called Conscious Dreaming. It is a strategy where you can connect to the abilities of your other aspects of self. Conscious Dreaming supports you in expanding your perceptual awareness, in connecting you to other dimensions of your self and the differing levels of your Higher Self. It exponentially expands us and all our abilites.

The tool is difficult to talk about, because it is a lot abstract. The more abstract an idea, concept or methodology, the more powerful it is for us to use. It takes us into the Truth of Who We Are as we surrender to it. The process is almost beyond description. I mean truly, how do we describe the splendor of Love, God, Life Everlasting and Eternality?

The other tool I wish to mention is connecting with your God Self to receive answers to all your questions. When you are ready and empty enough (when "your goblet has let go of enough old wine to create space for new wine and a new higher quality flavor, texture and bouquet"), then you will be ready to connect with your God Self.

There is no more powerful tool on the Earthplane at this time than connecting to your God Self. Why would we even want information from a lesser source, when we can get it directly from the Big Guy/ Lady ? When you endeavor to get in touch with your God Self and feel as though you have gotten nothing, it only means that you have more subconscious programming to release…more emptying to do. Do not despair. Keep on. At some point, you will have the door open to you. It is there for all of us, not just a precious few.

Our God Self will lovingly guide us every step of our Earthwalk as we are ready, willing to listen and take action with the recommendations given. With this open system of communication, we will have God at the helm with us in our waking and sleeping hours. We will have a wisdom and a compassion available to us that will raise our knowing and speed us into Union with the One.

35) MOVING WITH THE PARADIGM SHIFT

Let's face it, change is the only thing that is constant besides God's love for us. The paradigm is changing whether or not we want it to. Your participation will make the shift easier on you. Taxes and death are on their way out; they are a part of the old paradigm. God-Goddess never meant for us to be incarcerated in either of these inventions.

Our true nature is being restored to us thru Divine Intervention and the efforts of those awakening. We are speeding to the 100th monkey concept—to that magical 13 ½ %, where all of humanity who are ready and willing will make the leap into God consciousness in these bodies. Are you ready? Are you willing?

These bodies, the Living Temples of God will then be understood and aligned with continuous soulful decisions and actions. No longer will humanity behave like foolish mortals—bulletproof, unconscious in their decisions/actions, dishonoring both life and death.

There will be understanding that our bodies and the way we choose to live our lives is Spirit sent prayer and meditation. The old conditioned prayer beseeching God to forgive us as sinners, pathetic "poor me's" will be a memory of the past. No longer will we cling to our hope and faith as bouys in a raging ocean. We will live in certitude that we are God expressing always and command this is so consistently, to remind ourselves

As we recognize we are God expression in loving detachment continuously, we will realize that we are not here being judged by a fire and brimstone Master who we are subservient to; to whose call we must tow the line.

Our relationship with God will be different. It will be personalized, pleasing, easy and egalitarian. God is available to all of us just as She is available to Neale Donald Walsh, Ceanne DeRohan and a host of others.

Conversing with my God Self this a.m., I was told that I had it backwards. I am not here to have to please God. I am here to be God in enjoyment and amusement…that my relationship with God is totally based on this.

I also now have awareness that I am fulfilling my purpose, my higher purpose and following my highest desire. I am being responsible for my living temple and my life. I know how to respond to my emotional thoughts which create my body-mind-life experience. With my loving practices, I have this discipline. And because of this, I have risen victorious above senility and death. I know how to respond and am rising Goddess victorious now.

You have the same opportunity. It is why you are here now. Are you fulfilling your purpose, your higher purpose and following your highest desire? Do you know what they are?

Leonard Orr has been supporting humanity into this paradigm shift for the last 30 years. As the father of Conscious Energy Breathing/Rebirthing, he has personally trained hundreds of thousands of people around the globe to learn to breath energy as well as air. He has taught them to raise the quality of their emotional thoughts and their aliveness thru the sacred breath of life.

He has conquered eight terminal dis-eases in five years. He is the senility graduate par excellance. He has risen above senility and death and is filled with an energy, zest and enthusiasm for life that few people ever experience. He has risen above all the pretense of aliveness; above all the adrenalin induced states that most people rely on for their get up and go.

Leonard is a wise sage and a loving teacher. Spirit comes thru him in a marvelous way.

He has been writing prolifically these last few years as he is in constant communication with Source.

He is an enthusiastic advocate for people of all ages, in all walks of life all over the world. He is willing to be your personal friend. You must be sincere and genuine in your intent, because he can feel everything. There are not many teachers of Leonard's class that are available to the public and so approachable.

I highly recommend training with him at his training center in Virginia, USA. You will be changed forever. Go there open and humble. That is the only way we can learn anything. Being open and humble is the only way that our paradigm can shift within us.

36) WE ARE THE ONE GOD

Planet Earth has something like 6.4 billion God inhabiting it. Each of us was made in the image and likeness of our Divine Parents. As we awaken to the Truth of Who We Are thru whatever purification process (breath, Spirit, Will, prayer, meditation, processing, overcoming, etc.) we come into Union. The individuated beings we have been, have come to know, then, will reveal that there is only ONE MIND, ONE BODY, ONE AUTHORITY. And in this knowing, all Separation, blame, guilt, wrongful judgement cease to be.

Everything that existed without us (outside of us) is pulled within for rectification. All blaming others, all "look what you made me do", all anger at others, all fear of others, all feeling judged by others, all feeling criticized by others, all feeling condemned by others, all feeling rejected by others, all revenge for others, all feeling victim, abandonment and betrayal stops and changes. The finger pointing stops. Ownership begins and continues as we dismantle the conditioned emotional thoughts and experiences. Our tapes, programs change forever with our sincere intent and powerful tools.

Self blame, self anger, fear of the truth of who we are, self judgement, self criticism, self loathing, self condemnation, self rejection, self revenge, self abandonment, self betrayal are causal for the outpictures of our lives. As we work to undo these noxious misunderstandings, we get to a place within ourselves of doing this where we no longer blame ourselves nor beat ourselves up. We get to a place of guiltlessness, forgiveness, self acceptance, self love and understanding.

Remember: YOU HAVE NEVER, EVER DONE ANYTHING WRONG AND NEITHER HAS ANYONE ELSE AND UNTIL

YOU GET THIS, YOU WILL BE BLAMING SOMETHING, SOMEONE OR YOURSELF AND NOTHING HEALS.

There are times when some of us—God's workhorses feel dismayed, angry and overloaded with this Earth project of learning and healing our will—The Mother of Everything. And…we get to go higher and higher with our thought, feeling and energy because Mother Father God are pulling for us, dispensating us everyday. We just have to be willing to let them pull us into Union with Them. Don't abandon yourself. Renew yourself daily.

The opportunity to have a body to do this project is a highly sought after experience. There are literally hordes of disembodied energies/beings lusting after our experience. They want a body so badly…they see and know the opportunity. It is said that what is happening on the Earth right now is so auspicious an event, that formless beings are lined up with standing room only watching over us.

Remember, you need to be in body to achieve God consciousness. Don't blow it. Don't blow it off. Take advantage of the grace that has been given to you with and thru the beautiful body you have. And if it does not feel beautiful to you, you can melt off the "ugliness" thru all the healing modalities I have mentioned in this book. Remember, your thought-feeling is old conditioning that can change, if you want to change it.

It seems so crystal clear to me that the reason we are here is to realize our Divinity, to release, undo and revibrate our miscreated, misqualified energies—our conditioned emotional thoughts and to come into Union. Coming into Union does not mean that we all conform into the shape of a giant heart shaped cookie cutter. Coming into Union is recognizing and celebrating the Diversity of our Godhood and our humanity and our natural state.

Union is the pooling of all shapes, sizes, colors, designs, sounds into One Harmonious Cooperative Yummy Vibration. Union is acknowledging that your presence absolutely matters. **You Count Because You Are A Part Of The One**. God does not make mistakes. You are here because you are a part of the formula for success. You are part of the picture; what you do and say matters. You are contributory or you would not be here now. Do you get it?!

I knew before I was born that I desired to be here at this time. I demanded to be here. I wanted to be participatory in the most glorious experience this planet has ever known. My mother aborted me the first time I wanted to come in. So when I came in this last time, nothing was going to stop me. I came in with a very strong will—thanks to my mom's decision. (Thanks Mom.)

We all long for Union with God (with each other...that's why we always feel an emptiness). Most of us don't have a clue of what it is we feel we are missing. We just feel this emptiness, this lacking, this unfulfillment, this longing for "something'", THIS HOLE WITHIN OUR-SELVES. We search and search and search and experiment, experiment, experiment. "Is this what I'm looking for"? "Is this it"? This is what the quest for the Holy Grail is all about.

I long to come into complete Union with God-Goddess. I long to rise above all wrongful judgement, all misunderstanding, all misperception,, all miscreated, misqualified energy and experience. I long to be DIVINE TRUTH, DIVINE KNOWING, DIVINE WISDOM, DIVINE ONENESS. I long to transcend ordinary thought-feeling. For me being/having this would be Heaven on Earth and Everlasting Life.

I NOW CALL FORTH INTO THIS ETERNAL MOMENT OF NOW, I AM ONE WITH GOD–GOD-DESS IN HEAVEN ON EARTH IN THESE BODIES NOW. Mom and Dad, I am grateful that this is done.

I do not believe that we can speak about what Everlasting Life–Eternality is really, any more than we can concretize our thoughts about God, Source, Love and Truth. And our bodies know everything. What my body knows is that Eternity is who we are. We have always been and we will always be. And as I surrender my attachments to my form and all form of Creation, I will know an incomprehensible joy, bliss, serenity. And my body knows that it can know this and be this in this body-mind.

I have been working on "I AM Divine Patience". I ask all these questions and then ruminate over the status of my evolution and mankind's evolution into Godhood. When I am in ordinary reality, I feel desconsolate. When I am in extra-ordinary reality, in Higher Thought (thru the grace of the tools Source has granted me), I know without question that everyone, whether they are conscious of the evolutionary process of humanity into Godhood or not, are moving toward that goal. It is the destiny of this planet to do so.

The individuated experience is exquisitely unique for all of us as we move into our Godhood. Some of us will be asked to do what looks like more than others. Some of us will do what looks like less. Whatever it is, we signed on to do it or we would not be here now.

Some of you will be called upon to do senility. Know that you can survive it—if you want to. Know you can survive the death urge—if you want to. Know you can champion these conditions of the human experience—if you want to. Know you are Eternal and you can move into Life Everlasting past death and past old age. Know that you are very much a part of the Body-Mind-Spirit-Will of God. Know you are Divine. Know you do not need to kill your body to be in Heaven.

BE WILLING TO BE THE ETERNAL INSPIRATION AND EXPIRATION OF GOD-GODDESS IN HEAVEN ON EARTH IN THIS BODY-MIND IN THE PRESENT MOMENT OF NOW CONTINUOUSLY.

Jim Dvorak, Grand Master Quantum Dynamics Teacher says "The antidote to death is to keep breathing". (Thanks Jim!) Join me and others and be willing to keep breathing. Life is too happy to be short.

May God-Goddess speed you on your journey.

In Truth, Simplicity and Love,
Young Toni Delgado

POSTSCRIPT

All that exists is God. There is no thing that is not God. God is all inclusive. God is love, therefore everything is all inclusive in love. Every feeling, every emotion is a color vibration. Be willing to be the rainbow in Light. And consciously let go of the hard parts of the shadow.

Purify your love. Purify your Light. Cast out all doubt. You can remember your "Self". You have the ability to discern. Open to this ability now. You were created with a wonderful life force and aliveness. As you align with your will—your emotional body, you will raise your frequency—your color vibration into more aliveness; into your natural state of sentiency and connection to Source. Daily affirm the following as you use a delicious connected breath:

I now accept and choose to express my anger.
I now accept and choose to express my sadness.
I now accept and choose to express my resentments.
I now accept and choose to express my fear.
I now accept and choose to express my anxiety.
I now accept and choose to express my pain.
I now accept and choose to express my rage.
I now accept and choose to express my Light.

I gratefully cast out all guilt.
I gratefully cast out all blame.
I gratefully cast out all fault.
I gratefully cast out all hurt.
I gratefully cast out all kill.
I gratefully cast out all revenge.

I gratefully cast out all betrayal.
I gratefully cast out all darkness.

Jai! Victory to us One and All!

BIBLIOGRAPHY

Becker M.D., The Body Electric

Biser, Sam, Save your Life Videos

Bhartiji, The Vairagya Satakam

Castaneda, Carlos, Journey to Ixtlan, the Lessons of Don Juan; Tales of Power

Cota-Robles, Patricia Diane, What On Earth Is Going On?

The Course In Miracles

Delgado, Toni, Light Body Ascension Chart and Handbook
    Vol I Freeways to Higher Consciousness ebook
    Vol II Freeways to Higher Consciousness ebook
    Bursting the Body Light–Violet Flame of Forgiveness

DeRohan,Ceanne, The Right Use of Will; Original Cause

Guyton, Arthur P., Textbook of Medical Physiology

Hendricks, Gay, Conscious Breathing

Mails, Thomas, Frank Foolscrow; The Power and the Wisdom

Morter, Ted, Jr., D.C., The Healing Field

Prabhavananda, Swami and Manchester, Frederick The Wisdom of the Hindu Mystics, Upanishads, Breath of Life

Orr, Leonard, <u>Bhartriji</u>;
    <u>Breaking the Death Habit</u>;
    Conscious Connection, "The Death Urge"
    Turning Senility Misery Into Victory

Satprem, <u>On The Way To Supermanhood</u>

Schulze, Richard, <u>There Are No Incurable Dis-eases</u>

Skarin, Anna Lee, <u>Beyond Mortal Boundaries</u>

Spalding, Baird, <u>The Life and Teachings of The Masters of The Far East</u>

Walker, N.W. <u>Fresh Vegetable and Fruit Juices</u>

Watson, Lyall, <u>Gifts of Unknown Things</u>

Wright, Machaelle Small, <u>MAP: The Co-creativeWhite Brotherhood Medical Assistance Program</u>

For inquiries and loving support:

A Next Step…light center for emotional healing
Toni Delgado and Kelley Elkins
P.O. Box 429, Dona Ana, New Mexico 88032
www.anextstep.org toni@anextstep.org
505-382-8771

Leonard Orr
Rebirth International
Inspiration University
P.O. Box 1026, Staunton, VA. 24402
www.rebirthingbreathwork.com and **www.leonardorr.com**
rebirth @rica.com
540-885-0551

Dr. Richard Schulze
American Botanical Pharmacy
1-800-herbdoc (437-2362)

Sam Biser
Save Your Life Videos
1-800-485-5004

Patricia Diane Cota-Robles
The New Age Study of Humanity's Purpose
P.O. Box 41883
Tucson, Arizona 85717
www.1spirit.com/eraofpeace eraofpeace@aol.com

ABOUT THE AUTHOR

Toni Delgado resides in Las Cruces, New Mexico where she and her husband are A Next Step...light center for emotional healing. Toni trained and worked as a traditional psychotherapist, registered massage therapist and High School Instructor. She also trained and works as a Rebirther, Quantum Dynamics Teacher and Reiki Master. Toni is a Spiritual Healer and Earth Steward minister as well.

Toni believes mightily in the supreme regenerative capabilities of the body-mind and the triumph of the human spirit to supercede old conditioned belief systems. She also recognizes that humanity's return to Divinity is a must in our evolutionary process at this time and that it is happening and will continue to happen in spite of old conditioning.

0-595-24442-4